THE BIGGEST LOSER

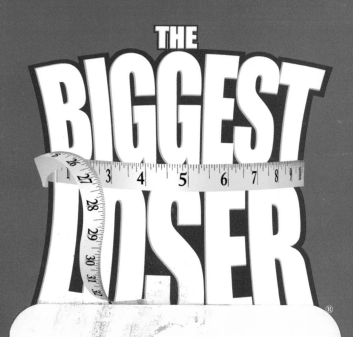

Q̲u̲i̲c̲k̲ & easy

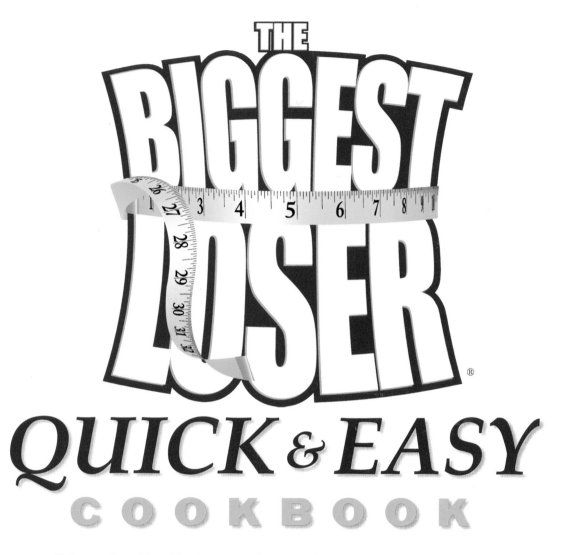

THE BIGGEST LOSER

QUICK & EASY COOKBOOK

Simply Delicious Low-Calorie Recipes to Make in a Snap

Chef Devin Alexander and *The Biggest Loser* Experts and Cast with Julie Will

Notice

This book is intended as a reference volume only, not as a medical manual. The information given here is designed to help you make informed decisions about your health. It is not intended as a substitute for any treatment that may have been prescribed by your doctor. If you suspect that you have a medical problem, we urge you to seek competent medical help.

The information in this book is meant to supplement, not replace, proper exercise training. All forms of exercise pose some inherent risks. The editors and publisher advise readers to take full responsibility for their safety and know their limits. Before practicing the exercises in this book, be sure that your equipment is well-maintained, and do not take risks beyond your level of experience, aptitude, training, and fitness. The exercise and dietary programs in this book are not intended as a substitute for any exercise routine or dietary regimen that may have been prescribed by your doctor. As with all exercise and dietary programs, you should get your doctor's approval before beginning.

Mention of specific companies, organizations, or authorities in this book does not imply endorsement by the author or publisher, nor does mention of specific companies, organizations, or authorities imply that they endorse this book, its author, or the publisher.

Internet addresses and telephone numbers given in this book were accurate at the time it went to press.

Rodale books may be purchased for business or promotional use or for special sales. For information, please write to: Special Markets Department, Rodale Inc., 733 Third Avenue, New York, NY 10017.

Printed in the United States of America
Rodale Inc. makes every effort to use acid-free ♾, recycled paper ♻.
Book design by Christina Gaugler
Illustration on page 13 by Judy Newhouse
Food photographs by Mitch Mandel/Rodale Images
Food styling by Diane Vezza and prop styling by Paige Hicks
All other photos by NBCUniversal Photo

Library of Congress Cataloging-in-Publication Data

Alexander, Devin.
    The Biggest loser quick and easy cookbook : more than 75 low-calorie and delicious meals in 20 minutes or less / Devin Alexander and the Biggest loser experts and cast.
        p.   cm.
    Includes index.
    ISBN 978–1–60961–423–2   paperback
    1. Quick and easy cooking.   2. Reducing diets—Recipes.   3. Biggest loser (Television program)   4. Cookbooks.
    I. Biggest loser (Television program)   II. Title.
    TX833.5.A43 2011
    641.5'55—dc23   2011036584

Distributed to the trade by Macmillan
2 4 6 8 10 9 7 5 3 1   paperback

 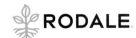 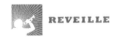

We inspire and enable people to improve their lives and the world around them.
www.rodalebooks.com

Production Development & Direction: Chad Bennett, Joni Camacho, Steve Coulter, Kim Niemi, Neysa Siefert

NBCU, Reveille, and 25/7 Productions would like to thank the many people who gave their time and energy to this project: Stephen Andrade, Carole Angelo, Sebastian Attie, Nancy N. Bailey, Alyssa Bieler, *The Biggest Loser* contestants, Dave Bjerke, Jill Bowles, Jill Carmen, Meegan Carroll, Scot Chastain, Ben Cohen, Jason Cooper, Marie Crousillat, Dr. Michael Dansinger, Kat Elmore, Cheryl Forberg, Devin Franchino, Jeff Friedman, Wendy Gable, Christina Gaugler, Marc Graboff, Bob Greenblatt, Jenny Groom, Bob Harper, Chris Harris, Paige Hicks, Shelli Hill, Susan Hindman, Dr. Robert Huizenga, Jill Jarosz, Helen Jorda, Edwin Karapetian, Alex Katz, Allison Kaz, Anna Kournikova, Loretta Kraft, Pam Krauss, Laura Kuhn, Beth Lamb, Todd Lubin, Roni Lubliner, Mitch Mandel, Rebecca Marks, Gregg Michaelson, Yelena Nesbit, Jessica Nubel, Julie Nugent, Kerry O'Donnell, Trae Patton, Ed Prince, Dolvett Quince, Scott Radloff, Joel Relampagos, Brandon Riegg, Karen Rinaldi, Melissa Roberson, Beth Roberts, Maria Rodale, Jessica Roth, Leslie Schwartz, Carrie Simons, Lee Straus, Kelia Tardiff, Paul Telegdy, Deborah Thomas, Julie True, Dianne Vezza, Emily Weber, Liza Whitcraft, Julie Will, Yong Yam

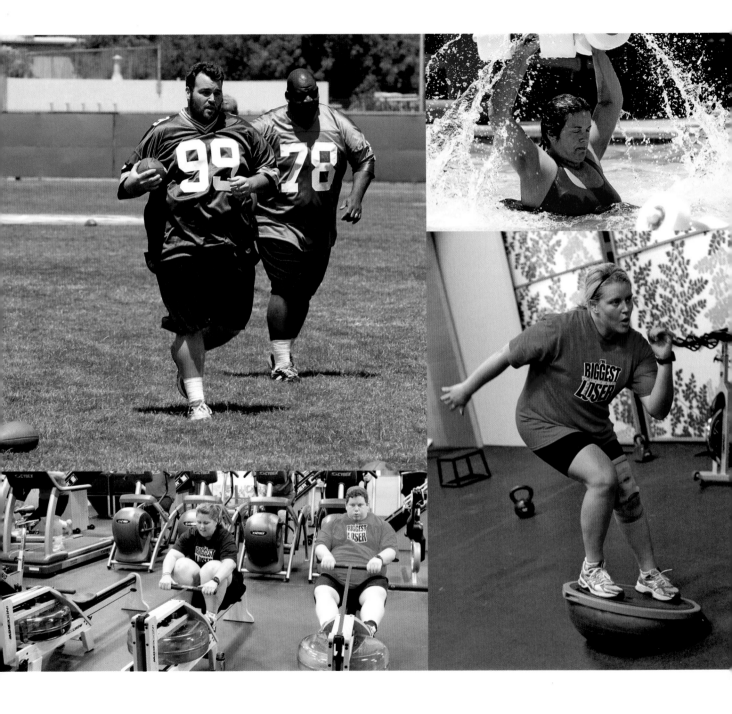

Contents

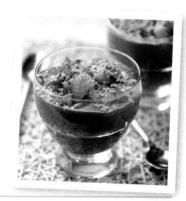

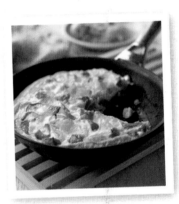

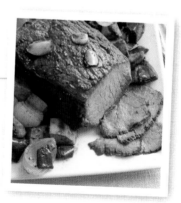

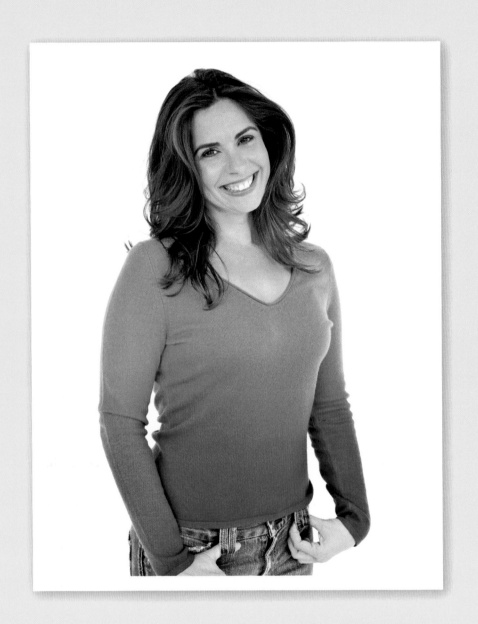

Introduction

I believe that one of the main reasons I've been able to maintain a 70-pound weight loss for close to 20 years is because I've learned to "be prepared" when it comes to food. The truth is, we're all insanely busy, and some days it just doesn't seem like there's enough time in the day to cook a healthy meal. So we grab something on the run that we know isn't great for us and, in many cases, doesn't even satisfy us. Then we're stressed out because we couldn't find time to burn those extra calories in the gym . . . and we come home exhausted yet again . . . and the cycle continues.

The next thing you know, you're writing to Bob, Anna, or even me saying, "Please help me. I'm so stuck. I just don't know what to eat!" But you probably do have a general sense of what to eat. You just don't know how to find the time to create a healthy eating plan without feeling overwhelmed.

Well, if you've opened up this book, you've taken the first step toward solving that problem. Over the years, I've tackled a wide variety of themes to help you create delicious, healthy food at home—from family-friendly, budget-conscious meals to guilt-free desserts to take-out favorites. And each time I traveled across the country to promote the books, speak to audiences, and give cooking demos, I heard the same response over and over: "Okay, now I believe that healthy food *can* taste great. I just don't have time to make it!"

Well, the excuses stop here. I promise you that you have enough time in your day to make the healthy meals and snacks in this book. I created these recipes with a wide variety of needs and occasions in mind. There are elegant dishes for entertaining (I always encourage people to bring their own healthy dishes to parties) like Asian Crab Salad–Topped Brown Rice Crisps (page 93) and Curry-Rubbed Pork Tenderloin with Peach Chutney (page 177), and happy hour faves like Sweet Potato No-Skins (page 94) and Pork Notsticker Lettuce Wraps (page 91). There are plenty of kid-friendly dishes that your whole family will love like Kids' Favorite Chicken "Pucks" (page 184) and Crustless Turkey "Pizza" (page 194). And there are tons of delicious, healthy options for quick and easy breakfasts, on-the-go lunches, simple dinners, and even snacks, desserts, and cocktails! Many of them can be packed for portable to-go meals that are way tastier and easier on your waistline than takeout. And unlike most "convenience options," they're all made with fresh, wholesome ingredients, so they're preservative free!

So the next time you think there just aren't enough minutes in the day to eat healthy, I suggest you flip through these pages and let your mouth start watering. You'll be shocked at how quickly you can throw together these satisfying, healthy dishes, many with as little as 5 to 10 minutes of prep time. Once you get into the habit of planning and packing your lunches and snacks like the *Biggest Losers* (and I) do, not only will you save money, you'll also find yourself eating more satisfying, delicious foods and still fitting into your favorite jeans.

It's truly an honor and a pleasure to be a part of *The Biggest Loser* community. I'm looking forward to hearing from each and every one of you—from your weight-loss struggles and successes, to your cooking challenges and concerns, to the recipes you want to see in future books!

Notes to the Chef, from the Chef

As is evident by the title, this book is all about making it a little easier to live a healthy lifestyle, no matter how much (or how little) time you have to spare each day. In the pages that follow, you'll find simple, delicious, calorie budget–friendly meals, snacks, and desserts that you can make in minutes—as well as tips and strategies from *The Biggest Loser* experts and contestants that will show you just how much of a difference 20 minutes a day can make in your weight-loss efforts.

Eating Clean

The Biggest Loser eating plan recommends an all-natural diet free of highly processed/refined foods, trans fats, preservatives, high-fructose corn syrup, and the artificial flavorings and sweeteners that are added to many "diet" foods to create flavor and texture. In my recipes, you will only find ingredients that follow those guidelines. (Per *Biggest Loser* expert Dr. Robert Huizenga's suggestion, I also avoided foods that contain evaporated cane juice, fructose, and many other ingredients that are often considered passable.)

In a perfect world, all of the experts on the show, myself included, strive toward eating a very clean diet of all-natural foods. That said, you have to create a sustainable weight plan that works for you and your family's needs. So if, as you start flipping through the recipes in this book, you think, "That sounds great, but I can't find that ingredient at my grocery store" or "I wonder if I can make this with the staples in my pantry, instead of investing in a whole new set of basics," don't worry. The guidelines in this book are just that—guidelines, not absolutes. The important thing is to create a healthy lifestyle that you can realistically adapt without feeling overwhelmed. You might start off by changing a few bad habits, and eventually eliminate most or all refined sugars or artificial ingredients from your diet—just as you might start your workouts 10 or 20 minutes at a time, and eventually build up to an hour or more. The keys to long-term weight loss are planning and consistency. Baby steps are okay.

I want to make it as easy for you as possible to enjoy the delicious recipes that I've developed for you in this book. To that end, I've compiled a list of ingredients that you might not be as familiar with, followed by a list of time-saving cooking strategies. I hope you'll peruse them before you get in the kitchen. I think they'll make grocery shopping and cooking a bit easier.

No-Sweat Shopping

I'd strongly encourage anyone trying to live a healthy lifestyle to visit a local natural food market or grocery store chain at least once a month.

There are so many new and interesting ingredients turning up on the shelves every day, many of which will become staples in your kitchen. If you can find a health food store that carries bulk foods in serve-yourself bins (many Whole Foods markets do), you can sample new ingredients without making a big up-front investment.

Take a trip to Whole Foods: Whole Foods Market is the world's largest retailer of natural and organic foods, with 200 stores throughout North America and the United Kingdom. It has a reputation for being a little pricey, and in some instances it can be (especially for specialty goods and organic produce), but I do believe that you can stock up on some basic staples there without breaking the bank. Whole Foods is great for buying products like infused olive oils, nitrate-free meats, low-sodium broths (as opposed to "lower sodium" found at many traditional grocery stores), salt-free spice blends, beans, and extra-healthy breads and tortillas, most of which have a long shelf life. Investing in a few good-quality oils and vinegars will pay off over time, and they will add a lot of flavor to the healthy dishes you create.

Shop in bulk: Another way to make shopping for natural foods more affordable is to buy in bulk. Peruse the bulk bins for grains like quinoa, oats, bulgur, and short-grain brown rice, as well as nuts, dried fruit, and other cooking essentials. Make an effort to plan ahead and shop smart, and I think you'll be pleasantly surprised by how much money you can save.

Key Ingredients

Below is a list of the key ingredients you'll need to make the recipes in this book, as well as suggested substitutes you can use in their place if you have trouble finding what the recipe calls for. Note that substitutions will affect the nutritional content and fat and calorie counts listed for each recipe, but they are still good options for health and weight management.

Almond Mozzarella Cheese

I was surprised by how much I enjoyed this naturally low-fat alternative to the dairy mozzarella cheese I used to rely on. While I won't pretend that it tastes like the "real thing," this cheese is really delicious and even melts like real mozzarella when heated in recipes like the Caprese Burger (page 116). I like the Lisanatti brand, which has only 50 calories and 1 gram of fat per ounce, making it 97 percent fat free. It also has 7 grams of protein per ounce and only 3 grams of carbohydrates. Lisanatti makes shredded almond mozzarella cheese, too, which may shave even more time off your cooking prep, so check your grocery store for that. If you can't find it, just purchase the lightest natural mozzarella cheese you can find instead.

Bagged Greens and Veggies

Mixed greens, spinach, arugula, and other lettuces are a great solution when you're tight on time (mostly because the majority of them have been triple washed, so you don't have to waste time washing and drying them). Most grocery stores also stock preshredded coleslaw mix, broccoli slaw mix, and bagged broccoli florets, all of which I've included in this book. No rinsing or picking is necessary. Simply cut open the bag and start cooking! Keep in mind that once these bags are opened, the remaining greens keep fresh longer if you leave the plastic unsealed and open in your fridge with plenty of room to "breathe." I'm not sure why most grocery clerks have a tendency to tightly close bags of produce as you're checking out (maybe to keep it from rolling around in your car), but keeping produce dry and in an open bag will help it last much longer.

Breads and Flatbreads

I know I'm going to start to sound like a broken record, but the most important thing when it comes to bread products is to read the labels. Buy any you like that has the least amount of preservatives and fat, and the most fiber you can find. Check the sodium and sugar, too. Some breads have way too much of both. I am currently a big fan of Julian Bakery's breads, particularly the Amazing Sourdough since it has only 60 calories per slice with

6 grams of fiber. I can make a big sandwich without a lot of calories. Sometimes I also use flatbreads for open-faced sandwiches, like in my Doctor Kracker Turkey Snacker (page 106). I love the hearty crispness of flatbreads. Doctor Kracker's are perfect because they're exactly 100 calories. Again, though, use any brand you can find that's healthy.

Cheese Spreads

In creating craveable wraps and sandwiches, I kept going back to spreadable low-fat cheeses and goat cheese as a way to make quick lunches that pack a lot of flavor without packing a lot of fat. I like the Alouette Light Garlic and Herbs Soft Spreadable Cheese as well as Chavrie with Basil and Roasted Garlic Goat's Milk Cheese spread, which was the perfect addition to my Herb Turkey Sandwich (page 123) because it packs such a huge amount of flavor. If you find other low-fat cheeses that look interesting, experiment away! Just make sure you choose spreads with no more than 50 calories and 3.5 grams of fat per 2-tablespoon serving. If you're having trouble finding either, you can always use a small amount of any goat cheese mixed with some fresh herbs or frozen herb cubes (see page xvi for more information).

Chicken and Seafood (Frozen)

Shrimp and other seafood will keep for a long time in the freezer, so you can buy these slightly more expensive products whenever you see them for a reduced price. Keep bags of frozen shrimp, langostinos (small lobsters), and flash-frozen fish fillets in your freezer so you can create a healthy fish dish anytime.

Note that if you are going to freeze chicken or fish, it's better to buy them frozen. If you buy fresh and then freeze these lean proteins, the quality will deteriorate since they were likely frozen before they were shipped to the store. If you refreeze and defrost them a second time, they are likely to lose flavor and texture.

Chocolate Chunks

It's no secret that I *love* chocolate! Like red wine, small amounts of dark chocolate have been linked to health benefits (like improving cardiovascular health) because they contain flavonoids, which are powerful antioxidants. In order to get these benefits, you must consume chocolate that is 70 percent or more pure cocoa, so make sure to check the label on your chocolate chunks or chocolate bar before you buy it. I keep coming back to all-natural 70 percent cocoa mini chocolate chunks because they're easy to find at my natural food market and make an excellent addition to dishes like Chocolate Raspberry Dreamers (page 204). If they're not easy to find at your market, just buy any dark chocolate bar or chocolate chips with at least 70 percent cocoa and chop them with a knife on your cutting board. Or stock up the next time you go to a natural food market, where they're sometimes sold in bulk as well as in bags. If you do buy them in bulk or open a package that you're not going to finish soon, be sure to store them in your freezer to keep them fresh for months. Plus, if you're anything like me, you're less likely to munch on them if they're tucked away in your freezer rather than sitting in your cabinet!

English Muffins and Hamburger Buns (Sprouted Grain and Whole Wheat)

Next time you're at the grocery store, consider taking a minute to read the labels of the "whole wheat" English muffins and bread products. You might be shocked by the number of preservatives, chemicals, and even sugars used in many brands. That said, without preservatives, these baked goods quickly get stale, so it can be hard to figure out the best option.

I use whole grain and sprouted grain English muffins for recipes that would generally call for English muffins. I also use them as hamburger buns in recipes like the Red, White, and Blue Burger (page 115). I searched high and low for 3½-inch-diameter all-natural, whole grain, low-fat hamburger buns that actually tasted half as good as traditional hamburger buns. If they exist, I could not find them. A great substitute is Rudi's Organic Bakery Whole Grain Wheat English Muffins. They're a bit higher in calories than what I

would prefer to use for a burger or sandwich, but they contain 3 grams of fiber and don't taste "healthy," which is so important to me—I find it's easier to eat healthy when you feel like you're indulging. They're also much softer than many whole grain buns, mimicking that pleasing texture of many processed breads. There are some all-natural hamburger buns available that are pretty good (though I like Ezekiel's Sprouted Grain English Muffins over their hamburger buns, even for hamburgers!), but keep in mind that they're probably bigger than the 3½-inch-diameter size I recommend. You can cut the larger ones to size and freeze the scraps for homemade bread crumbs.

Flavored Extra-Virgin Olive Oils

You'll notice that several recipes in this book call for flavored olive oils, such as Meyer lemon-infused extra-virgin olive oil in the Lemon Arugula Salad (page 139) and jalapeño lime-infused extra-virgin olive oil in the Fresh-As-Can-Be Jalapeño Lime Scallops (page 196). These ingredients might sound a bit intimidating or pricey, but a little truly goes a long way. They add a depth of flavor to dishes that I think makes them well worth the extra investment. I also think flavored oils make fantastic host gifts. Instead of buying a $15 bottle of wine that someone will enjoy only once, get him or her a bottle of flavored olive oil (O Olive Oil, www.ooliveoil.com, sells many varieties for less than $20) and tuck it into a wine gift bag. Your host will think of you everytime he or she uses it.

Herb Cubes (Frozen)

Frozen cubes of prechopped herbs are becoming widely available at many grocery stores. I recommend stocking your freezer with the basil, cilantro, and ginger varieties. They'll save you tons of time since you won't need to wash or chop the herbs. And they'll potentially even save you money because you can use only what you need and keep the remainder frozen for months. You simply pop out one cube at a time and defrost it. The brand I see most often in stores is Dorot. Search your store's freezers to see what you can find. Just be sure to choose a brand that is preservative free.

The one exception for me is garlic. Nothing can replace the flavor of freshly chopped garlic, especially in dishes like the Pork Notsticker Lettuce Wraps (page 91).

Ketchup and BBQ Sauce (Low Sugar/Low Sodium)

These days, you can find several options of both of these sauces widely available at many grocery store chains, so it's just a matter of finding a brand you like. Note that some ketchups and barbecue sauces might not be marked "low sodium" or "low sugar," so you'll need to read labels and compare to find ones that aren't too high in salt or sugar. If possible, it's better to select a brand that is sweetened with honey or agave nectar, which have lower glycemic index values than sweeteners like cane juice or sugar.

Lemon and Lime Juice

It's very tempting to depend on bottled lemon and lime juices, but for the sake of your food and your tastebuds, please don't succumb to these grocery store traps. I promise that it won't break your time budget to squeeze juice from whole lemons and limes—and it's so worth it. If you don't believe me, do a taste test for yourself. Pour a bit of bottled lemon or lime juice on a teaspoon and taste it. Then do the same with the fresh. I'll be shocked if you ever turn back. Oh, and if you store your lemons and limes in the refrigerator, they'll last much longer than keeping them in the fruit bowl on your counter.

Marinara Sauce

A jar of ready-to-go marinara sauce is super helpful for quick and easy dinners, but you have to be very mindful of the fat and calorie contents. Read the labels on jarred sauces at the store (I once found an "organic," "natural" sauce that had 13 grams of fat per ½-cup serving—yikes!) and experiment until you find one that you love. I love the taste of Monte Bene Tomato Basil Pasta Sauce, which manages to be low fat and low salt, without any added sugar, and it is still delicious!

Mayonnaise

For truly delicious, moist burgers and sandwiches that don't taste at all like "diet" food, I use Spectrum Naturals Light Canola Mayo, which is an all-natural, reduced-fat sandwich spread. It has only 3.5 grams of fat per tablespoon, 0 grams of saturated fat, and only 65 milligrams of sodium, with no preservatives, sugar, or artificial ingredients. And it happens to be eggless and vegan, which is a plus for some. Feel free to swap in any brand with similar nutritional value if you have trouble finding that one. I also used a lemon-flavored reduced-fat mayo, The Ojai Cook Lemonaise Light, in my Lobster Slaw Salad (page 133). If you can't find that, you can use any other reduced-fat lemon-flavored mayonnaise. Or, in a pinch, I sometimes use the Spectrum Naturals and add a bit of fresh lemon juice and True Lemon dehydrated lemon powder.

Packaged Meats

The good news when it comes to deli meats and bacon is that nitrate- and nitrite-free meats are more widely available than ever before. I recently noticed that Safeway started stocking all-natural meats under its own label, called Open Nature. That means that major grocery store chains are hearing and fulfilling your requests for healthy and preservative-free options. In addition, many other major brands are offering nitrate-free versions of their top sellers. Just be sure to read the nutrition labels carefully for fat and saturated fat content. There are still a lot of chicken and turkey sausages and bacons out there that have a ton of fat. I use the Applegate Organics brand often because it tends to be the leanest, and I really like the taste of all of their products that I've tried. (That said, I think their turkey salami tastes more like bologna than traditional Italian salami, but I really don't have a problem with that, especially since their turkey bologna contains significantly more fat, as do other brands).

Quinoa

I see quinoa popping up on more and more restaurant menus lately, which is great because it's a very healthful seed that, unlike wheat or oats, has about 12 to 18 percent protein content. It looks almost like a seed when coming from a box, but it becomes fluffy when cooked and has a slightly nutty flavor. Whether you try it hot for breakfast in my Buff Blueberry Quinoa (page 80) or as an amino acid–rich side dish in my Gazpacho Quinoa (page 142), I hope you find quinoa to be as yummy as I do. If you cook up a big batch on the weekend, you can keep it in the fridge and add it to dishes all week long.

Raita, Salsas, and Other Sauces

Since this cookbook is written for time-crunched people (aren't we all?), I've included a number of dishes that you can throw together with a little help from delicious prepared sauces. For example, my Super Simple Slaw (page 148) is simply bagged broccoli slaw tossed with a store-bought Indian-inspired raita dip. It's a fantastic time-saver to use sauces like these, but it's essential to carefully read the labels on raita, salsa, Indian simmer sauce, olive tapenade, pesto, and any other prepared sauces you buy. Always look at the calories, fat, saturated fat, and sodium per serving. Check the serving size, too—sometimes it is unrealistically small, and the idea is to save time in the kitchen, not add time to your gym schedule!

If you have trouble finding any of the sauces suggested for the recipes in this book, feel free to substitute. For the raita dip, consider another natural yogurt-based dip or salad dressing that you'd likely find in the refrigerator section near the produce at the grocery store. For the Indian simmer sauce, just take a stroll down the international aisle. A good Korean barbecue sauce would work well if you're in the mood for a different flavored simmer (just make sure it doesn't have an astronomical amount of sodium). It's more important to focus on the healthy cooking techniques in the recipes than on any one specific product.

Salad Dressings

There are many brands of reduced-calorie and reduced-fat dressings on the market these days, but buyer beware: Low-fat and fat-free salad dressings are commonly filled with chemicals and preservatives (such as MSG) and tons of sugar. That said, you can definitely find brands that are all natural. A couple of my favorites are Follow Your Heart Lowfat Ranch Dressing and Bolthouse Farms Creamy Italian Dressing. Remember to always check labels for added sugars and be mindful of the sodium content in bottled dressings.

Salt-Free Seasoning Blends

Admittedly, it can be a challenge to create flavorful dishes that are low in fat and low in sodium. I've always liked using salt-free seasonings to help boost flavor without relying on salt. That said, I wasn't fully aware of the scope of varieties now available until recently. Of course, Mrs. Dash has some great ones, but other brands, such as The Spice Hunter, also offer some incredible salt-free blends that make healthy cooking so much quicker and easier. Their chili powder blend made for an extremely simple to make, yet complex seeming Chili-Rubbed London Broil (page 166). Their curry blend helped create the Curry-Rubbed Pork Tenderloin with Peach Chutney (page 177), which is impressive enough to serve to your mother-in-law, a date, or your boss. I also use their mesquite blend, Cajun Creole blend, and garlic herb bread blend in this book. If you can't find these spices easily, it might be worth ordering them online. If you don't want to do that, you can swap in any other similar natural rub. Just be sure to read labels. Many rubs have sugar and salt in them, and in many cases, that's one of the first ingredients on the label (which means it contains more sugar or salt than any other ingredient—not a good thing).

Tortillas (Sprouted Grain and Whole Spelt)

I don't tend to be a fan of most sprouted grain tortillas—they are better for you, but usually taste "better for you," if you know what I mean. But I was excited to find a sprouted-grain tortilla from French Meadow Bakery at Whole Foods that has a pleasant "chewy" texture like tortillas are supposed to have (not the stale texture that many sprouted grain breads tend to have). If you can't find those or another brand of sprouted grain tortillas that you love, whole spelt tortillas are my second choice. (I love Rudi's Organic Bakery; make sure you're buying "whole spelt" and not just "spelt.") Whole spelt tortillas are great because they tend to taste nearly as decadent as other store-bought tortillas, yet have considerably

less fat and sodium than other natural varieties. If you can't get either easily, just compare all of the brands at your store. Go with one that is about 8 inches in diameter and around 120 to 150 calories. You'll note that I suggest sprouted grain in all recipes using a tortilla throughout the book as a first choice except in the Sooo Not Chicken Nuggets (page 107). When made with a spelt or more traditional tortilla, they really taste like chicken nuggets. But when made with a sprouted grain tortilla, they just don't taste like the real thing.

You'll see that I often call for "10-inch sprouted grain tortilla or 8-inch whole spelt." That's because the 10-inch sprouted grain has about the same number of calories as the 8-inch whole spelt and no additional fat.

Veggies (Frozen)

Most frozen veggies are picked at the peak of freshness and are minimally processed, making them a perfect, all-natural time-saver. Peruse the frozen section at the grocery store to see what options are available. It's smart to have a bag of frozen peppers and onions on hand for my Sausage Feta Pepper Bake (page 72)—prechopped veggies will definitely save you a ton of time. Specialty veggies like artichoke hearts can be a bit expensive, so grab them when you see them on sale.

Time-Saving Tips

Nonstick Foil

This cookbook is meant to free you from slaving over the stove, but that doesn't mean you should have to slave over the sink, either! I encourage you to line your baking sheets and roasting pans with nonstick foil (or parchment) so that cleaning up is as painless as possible. Make sure you use foil (as opposed to parchment paper) for oven temperatures of more than 400°F, as paper can catch fire at higher temps!

Garlic Cloves

While I do recommend that you mince your own fresh garlic in all recipes, you can save time by buying the pre-peeled cloves. If you cook often, they're no more costly than regular heads of garlic. Look for pre-peeled cloves in the produce section, often near bagged lettuces or packaged herbs.

Food Processors and Blenders

A good food processor will make for a frustration-free time in the kitchen when you're in a hurry. A food processor is super handy for quickly chopping the fresh veggies in recipes like Gazpacho Quinoa (page 142), instead of laboring over a cutting board. A good-quality blender with an ice-crush setting is essential for making healthy smoothies and drinks, like my Punched-Up Piña Colada (page 213). If you make frozen drinks often, you might want to consider investing in a blender that has a food processor attachment, like a Cuisinart SmartPower Deluxe Blender/Food Processor, a two-in-one appliance that will save you money and precious counter space in smaller kitchens.

To-Go Containers

If you take the time to pack your food for breakfast or lunch on the go, you'll never get stuck with unhealthy options on the road. Many of the recipes in this book can travel with you, so investing in a couple of quality resealable plastic containers that you can take to work every day is a good idea. Some companies even make containers with compartments so you can pack salads that will stay crisp and fresh instead of becoming wilted and soggy. Oggi Corporation makes a Chill-To-Go Food Container with a fork, spoon, and removable freezer pack all in one (available online at retailers such as amazon.com or opensky.com). It's perfect for dishes like the Watermelon Feta Salad (page 137), since you want to separate the watermelon chunks from the salad greens, cheese, and shrimp, while keeping the dressing in its own container. Then, come lunchtime, you can easily assemble a restaurant-quality salad in seconds.

Cooler

Depending on the length of your commute or daily drive to work, you may want to invest in a cooler to keep your meals at food-safe temperatures. Coleman even makes coolers that you can plug in to your car's cigarette lighter and then plug in to the outlet in your office, so you can keep your food cold for a long time. They're also great for making sure your family eats healthy on road trips and will keep you from diving into the minibar in the hotel room because you were "starving."

Stock Up

When you get home late and have to put dinner on the table in a snap, it's really useful to have a well-stocked pantry full of healthy, delicious ingredients that can be thrown into a meal at a moment's notice. As previously noted, keeping your freezer stocked with healthy proteins and vegetables is a must. Other options—like cans of low-sodium, water-packed tuna and the crabmeat found in the refrigerated section of your grocery store (in sealed cans)—are also great to have on hand. Cans of crabmeat can last quite a long time in your refrigerator. Stock up on a couple of cans and you can whip up my Asian Crab Salad–Topped Brown Rice Crisps (page 93) for your hungry family or last-minute guests in no time. Also keep your pantry stocked with healthy grains and sauces like couscous (which takes only 5 minutes to cook), brown rice crisps, brown rice cakes, whole wheat pastas, and marinara sauce.

Martini Glasses

As I always tell *The Biggest Loser* contestants, we eat with our eyes first, so it really helps to have a few great presentation pieces in your cupboard. Simple martini glasses are great for serving my Watermelon Cocktail (page 211) and many other foods for a pretty presentation.

Quick and Easy Basics

Knowing how to cook these two healthy staples will shave prep time from your evening meal routine. I recommend keeping grilled chicken and prepared quinoa in the fridge at all times so that you can whip up healthy breakfasts, lunches, and dinners in mere minutes without starting from scratch.

ESSENTIAL GRILLED CHICKEN

Any good cookbook author knows not to repeat recipes from book to book. That said, it is virtually impossible to write a healthy cookbook without a recipe for Basic Grilled Chicken (as I called a similar recipe in my book The Most Decadent Diet Ever!*) or Simple Grilled Chicken (as I called it in* The Biggest Loser Family Cookbook*). Truth is, this recipe simply is essential. I love to keep grilled chicken on hand for salads, sandwiches—even pizzas.*

4 (4-ounce) boneless, skinless chicken breasts, visible fat removed

Olive oil spray (propellant free)

Salt, to taste

Fresh ground black pepper, to taste

Preheat a grill to high heat.

Lightly mist both sides of each chicken breast with the olive oil spray. Sprinkle them lightly with salt and then pepper. Grill for 3 to 5 minutes per side, or until no longer pink. Serve immediately.

Makes 4 servings

Per serving: **127 calories, 26 g protein, 0 g carbohydrates (0 g sugar), 2 g fat, trace saturated fat, 66 mg cholesterol, 0 g fiber, 74 mg sodium**

BASIC QUINOA

Only a few years ago, most Americans had never heard of quinoa. But these days, it's not hard to find in grocery stores and on restaurant menus across the country. And that's a great thing since this versatile grain is high in protein and contains all eight essential amino acids.

You know that quinoa is fully cooked when the grains become transparent and their spiral-like germs "pop" out. If you are new to quinoa, try it out in a sweet bowl of Buff Blueberry Quinoa (page 80) or use it in a salad with a lot of bold flavors.

---

2 cups water

1/4 teaspoon salt

1 cup white quinoa

Pour the water in a medium nonstick pot and place it over high heat. When the water boils, add the salt and quinoa. Cover the pot and reduce the heat. Simmer for 14 to 16 minutes, or until all of the water is absorbed.

Makes 4 (3/4-cup) servings

Per serving: **180 calories, 7 g protein, 29 g carbohydrates (2 g sugar), 4 g fat, 0 g saturated fat, 0 mg cholesterol, 11 g fiber, 155 mg sodium**

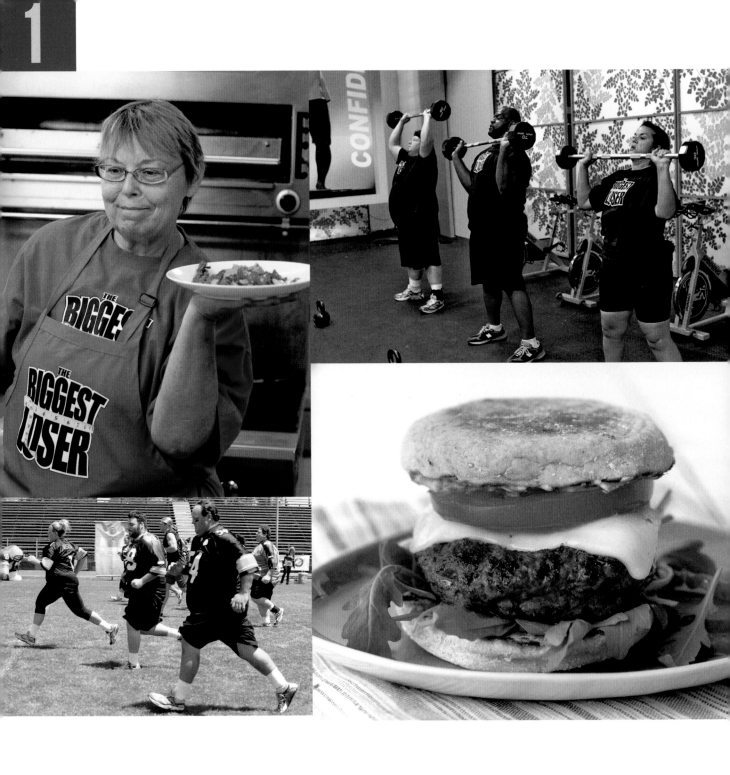

The Biggest Loser Eating Plan

"I wish I could, but I just don't have the time."

These days, It's become an all-too-common refrain. Whether we're talking about going to the grocery store, cooking healthy meals, working out, or simply sitting down to the dinner table with our families, most of us have such busy schedules that it can feel impossible to carve out any time for a healthy lifestyle.

Why are we so busy all the time? Well, for starters, many Americans are feeling the pressure to work longer hours than ever before to pay for the rising costs of living expenses, to save for retirement, or simply to ensure that they keep their jobs. Between working and caring for our families, many of us feel too exhausted or stressed out at the end of the day to even think about cooking dinner or consider going to the gym.

But when we don't take the time to take care of ourselves, we're not conserving our time or our money. As we all know by now, obesity is closely linked to many life-threatening diseases, such as type 2 diabetes, high blood pressure, heart disease, and some cancers. When we don't nourish our bodies with wholesome foods, get enough sleep, and stay active, we put ourselves at an elevated risk for developing health problems that are expensive to treat and can not only diminish the quality of our lives, but take years off of them.

In the pages that follow, you'll learn the basics of *The Biggest Loser* eating plan and exercise guidelines. While sustainable weight loss is a slow and steady process that requires hard work and discipline, just 20 minutes a day can make a real difference in your overall health. Sure, there will be days when the thought of making dinner feels too overwhelming. That's why Chef Devin has provided meal ideas you can throw together in just a few minutes, with a little planning ahead. When you map out a week's worth of meals in advance, shop accordingly on the weekends, and keep your refrigerator stocked with healthy ingredients, "not enough time" will no longer be an excuse to eat poorly.

Think about it: In less than 20 minutes a day, you can change the quality of your life. You're worth the investment.

Counting Calories

Yes, it's important to count calories. Why? Because one pound is made of 3,500 calories, and in order to shave off some pounds, you have decrease the amount of calories you take in through food and increase the amount of calories you burn through exercise.

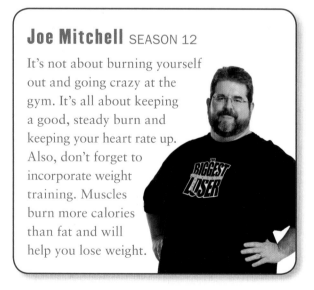

Joe Mitchell SEASON 12

It's not about burning yourself out and going crazy at the gym. It's all about keeping a good, steady burn and keeping your heart rate up. Also, don't forget to incorporate weight training. Muscles burn more calories than fat and will help you lose weight.

A calorie is a measurement of how much energy the food you eat provides for your body. You need energy to fuel physical activity as well as all metabolic processes, from maintaining your heartbeat to digesting your meals. Only four components of the food you eat supply calories: protein and carbohydrates (4 calories per gram), alcohol (7 calories per gram), and fat (9 calories per gram). Vitamins, minerals, fiber, and water do not contain calories.

Keep in mind that the quality of the calories you eat is just as important as the quantity you take in. Some calories provide fuel for your workouts, keep you feeling energized, and help your body stay healthy. Other calories (often referred to as "empty calories") don't really provide any benefits—in fact, they can make you feel tired, sluggish, and hungrier than you were before you ate. *The Biggest Loser* plan will show you how to fuel your body with the nutrients and energy it needs to lose weight and maintain overall health.

Season 5's Neill Harmer says he likes to think of calories as a daily allowance. "Let's say you have 2,000 calories to spend per day. If you drink that iced latte with whipped cream and chocolate, you just spent a BIG part of your allowance on something that really wasn't needed. Spend calories wisely."

The Biggest Loser plan helps you determine the exact calorie intake you require to meet your individual weight-loss goals. If you weigh 150 pounds or more, the simple calculation below will allow you to determine how many calories you should aim to eat each day. If you weigh less than 150 pounds, talk to a doctor about an appropriate calorie budget for your needs.

Calorie Budget:

**Your present weight × 7 =
total daily calorie budget**

As you lose weight, you'll need to continually reassess and reduce your calorie budget, in order to keep losing weight and break through plateaus. As you know from watching the show, *The Biggest Loser* contestants lose a lot of weight during their first few weeks at the Ranch. But after they've been at the Ranch for a little while and have less weight left to lose, they must readjust their calorie budgets and increase the intensity and duration of their workouts to keep losing.

All of the contestants have a daily homework assignment: At the end of the day, they tally up the total number of calories they consumed throughout the day. If they ate more calories than their budget calls for, it's up to them to burn off the extra calories by getting in one last workout, going for a walk, or doing a few laps in the pool.

Planning Your Calories

Once you've determined your daily calorie budget, the next step is to plan your meals and snacks accordingly. On *The Biggest Loser* plan, it's recommended that you eat three meals and two snacks each day. Parceling out your calories throughout the day ensures that you'll stay full and keep your blood sugar level stable. It will also prevent you from feeling deprived, keep you energized for exercise, and help you establish a regular pattern of eating that helps counter impulse eating and bingeing.

"At first, I had to work to get all of my meals in," recalls Season 8 winner Danny Cahill. "I wasn't used to eating healthy foods, but I quickly realized that nutritious food was way more satisfying than the fast food I had been eating. Eating healthy throughout the day kept my energy level up, and I felt fueled for my workouts."

Use the simple calculations below to determine how to best allocate your calorie budget throughout the day. In this example, the calorie budget is 1,800—yours may be more or less, depending on your goal and starting weight.

Calorie Budget = 1,800

1,800 / 4 = 450

450 / 2 = 225

So for each meal—breakfast, lunch, and dinner—the calorie budget is 450. For each snack, the calorie budget is 225.

This calculation is just a starting point. You

can create any distribution of calories that works for you and keeps you feeling satisfied. Season 5 winner Ali Vincent has a strategy that works for her: "I always eat within half an hour of waking up to jump-start my metabolism. Then I eat every 3 to 4 hours, be it a meal or a snack. I think this is just as important for me as exercise," she says.

If you go to the gym in the morning and require a bigger breakfast to fuel your workout, feel free to shift your calorie load toward the beginning of the day. Or if you work out just before dinner, you might want to have a bigger snack before the gym and a smaller dinner afterward. Create a distribution of calories that works for you. The important thing is to plan ahead and stay within your calorie budget. As Season 7's Nicole Brewer wisely advises, "Planning will save you. Prepare your snacks and meals ahead of time, and always have them with you."

To understand your body's hunger signals and how to interpret them, see *The Biggest Loser* Hunger Scale on the opposite page.

Planning Meals and Snacks

As Nicole says, planning is an essential component of successful weight loss. The times when you are likely to be the most tempted to stray from your calorie budget are those when you're caught without a good option. In other words, when you've failed to plan, you've planned to fail.

Think about the week ahead each Sunday. Are there a few nights that you anticipate being too busy to cook? The recipes in this book give you many quick, delicious options for meals and snacks that you can take on the go, so plan ahead and cook several meals at once. Then store individual portions in resealable containers that you can heat up as needed.

When it comes to snacks, make sure you always have healthy choices readily available. Season 6's Ed Brantley says he keeps hard-boiled

Becky Comet SEASON 12

Find a workout buddy who can keep going even when you don't feel like it—and you can do the same for them. Then, afterward, you and your workout buddy can celebrate your successes together. Find someone who won't take your excuses (and you won't take theirs). At the Ranch, there were times when I didn't really feel like working out. But I had teammates who would tell me to get to the gym with them. Sometimes all I needed was an encouraging word.

The Biggest Loser Hunger Scale

1. **Famished or starving:** You feel weak and/or lightheaded. This is a big no-no.

2. **Very hungry:** You can't think of anything else but eating. You're cranky and irritable and can't concentrate.

3. **Hungry:** Your stomach's growling and feels empty.

4. **A little bit hungry:** You're just starting to think about your next meal.

5. **Satisfied:** You're comfortable, not really thinking about food. You feel alert and have a good energy level.

6. **Fully satisfied:** You've had enough to eat, maybe a little too much. Maybe you took a few extra bites for taste only, not hunger.

7. **Very full:** Now you need to unzip your jeans. You're uncomfortable, bloated, tired. Maybe you don't feel great. Where's the couch . . . ? You should never feel like this after a meal.

HUNGER SCALE FLASH CARD

1–3: Eat! Eat!

5: Stop, especially if you're trying to lose weight.

6: Definitely stop.

7: You may have waited too long. Better go find the couch and start over tomorrow.

If your hunger is anywhere from level 1 through 3, you should eat.

If you're at level 4, drink a glass of water, chew a piece of sugar-free gum, or do something else to distract yourself from thinking about food.

When you're trying to lose weight, you should try to stop eating when you reach level 5, but definitely no later than level 6. If you get to level 7, you've eaten too much. Anything above that is way too much and will sabotage your weight-loss efforts.

eggs and baggies of fresh-cut fruit in his fridge at all times, so he has healthy options when hunger strikes, and he can easily take them on the road.

Breakfast

If you haven't typically been a breakfast eater, you may struggle with the idea of eating within an hour of waking up—but it's essential that you do so. Try starting small and eating something simple, like some whole grain toast with almond butter or oatmeal with fruit. Eventually, you can work your way up to heartier breakfasts like Chef Devin's Asparagus and Chicken Apple Sausage Scramble (page 71) or Steak and Egg Breakfast Bowl (page 75).

Season 11's Austin Andrews says he's always loved eating breakfast—sometimes a little too much for his own good. His favorite dishes were carb-heavy meals like buttermilk pancakes or French toast with maple syrup and butter. These days, he still eats a hearty morning meal, but he's made some important swaps. Instead of eating a plate full of empty calories that would leave him hungry by mid-morning, he eats a breakfast that fuels him until lunchtime. "These days, I make French toast with whole wheat bread instead of white, and top it with fresh strawberries and a little stevia instead of high-calorie syrup. It's absolutely delicious."

Season 10 winner Patrick House says he usually eats a protein-heavy breakfast to keep him feeling satisfied throughout the morning. "I like to eat egg whites and turkey bacon or ham on an English muffin," he says. "I also eat some fruit, and I always have a glass of milk in the morning."

No matter what kind of a breakfast eater you are, "not enough time" in the morning is not an excuse to skip this important meal.

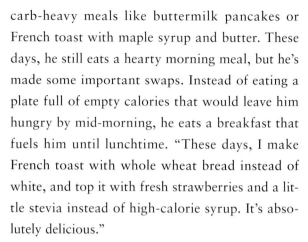

Shay Sorrells
SEASON 8

I used to love great family-style southern breakfasts. Now I use one whole egg and add egg whites for my scrambled eggs. I use turkey bacon instead of the real stuff, and I use Ezekiel raisin bread for toast. I substitute some fresh fruit for potatoes.

Lunch

When you're running around between school activities, appointments, or meetings, it can be very tempting to grab lunch from a drive-thru or a vending machine. After all, who has time to actually sit down and eat lunch during the week?

Well, you do. Everyone has 15 minutes to sit down and eat a healthy lunch. Doing so will help keep your metabolism on an even keel for the rest of the day.

Make sure your lunch includes a combination of lean protein, complex carbs, and healthy fats. You might have a salad with lots of vegetables and a serving of lean protein, or a sandwich made with whole grain bread. Danny Cahill says he's discovered an easy lunch that contains all of the nutrients he needs to keep up his energy for the afternoon. "Turkey bacon is one of the most amazing foods I discovered on the Ranch!" he raves. "It's so satisfying. I can whip up a quick lunch with a whole wheat tortilla, turkey bacon, and freshly chopped veggies and tomato. I'm ready to go in 5 minutes."

You've got a lot to accomplish in your afternoon, so feed yourself wisely!

Snacks

You should plan to eat your snacks mid-morning and mid-afternoon, a few hours after you've eaten breakfast or lunch and/or when you're beginning to feel hungry or tired. As a general rule, snacks should be eaten about every 3 to 4 hours, which will help keep cravings at bay and keep your energy up so that you feel alert and focused.

Aim for a snack that combines a serving of carbohydrates (such as a piece of whole fruit) with a half-serving of protein (such as a piece of low-fat cheese). Protein will help you feel full and satisfied, and when combined with carbs, a snack will help to keep your blood sugar stable.

Season 10's Lisa Mosely says she's learned that sometimes the simplest snacks are the most deli-

Courtney Rainville
SEASON 12

Keep focusing on the end result—what you'll look like, how you'll feel, that you'll be an athlete. Imagine that to push yourself through your workouts.

cious. "You don't always have to cook to eat," she says. "Make something out of the healthy ingredients in your fridge in seconds." She suggests a mid-morning snack of lean turkey tucked into lettuce leaves. "It's so quick and healthy."

One of Lisa's favorite afternoon snacks includes a few whole grain crackers with garlic hummus. "Before, I used to snack on potato chips. But now, these are like having a treat. I love that great crunch and salt combination," she says, "plus I get protein from the chickpeas in the hummus."

Dinner

Take the time to slow down and enjoy your dinner. It doesn't have to be your biggest meal of the day. In fact, Trainer Bob Harper advises contestants to eat "lean and green" at night and avoid carbohydrate-heavy meals. For the contestants at the

Ranch, dinner preparations are usually pretty simple. They might throw together a fresh salad with some grilled chicken or shrimp, or heat up some soup.

Season 11's Irene Alvarado says she used to sit down to a hearty, rich, protein-heavy meal at the end of the day. Today she still enjoys a satisfying evening meal, but she's changed her choice of protein. "I now appreciate lean cuts of meat like filet mignon," she says. "I just add a little seasoning and grill, and I'm good to go."

Season 11 winner Olivia Ward says that she and her sister, Season 11 finalist Hannah Curlee, used to make a quick seafood dinner on the Ranch. "We loved to grill cod with a little bit of lemon juice and fresh dill. We'd grill the fish for a couple of minutes on each side. Just before it was done cooking, we'd brush it with a teaspoon of wasabi mustard for a little bit of kick. It's very zippy! Have it with some broccoli or greens. Dinner!"

Joe Mitchell SEASON 12

Keep your goals in front of you. Use an erasable marker and write all your goals on your bathroom mirror. It will wipe off easily, so you can always update your goals and make new ones.

With mouthwatering, under-20-minute meals like Grilled Buffalo Steak with Horseradish Cream (page 172), Cranberry Goat Cheese Chicken (page 181), and Chicken and Shells in Vodka Sauce (page 187), you're sure to find the time to squeeze dinner into your busy schedule.

Write It Down

Though the contestants are required to keep a journal of the foods they eat each day at the Ranch, maintaining a food journal is one habit that most *Biggest Losers* will tell you they can't live without, even long after they've gone home.

Once your daily calorie budget is established, record your food and beverage intake daily. You can use the Sample Food Journal page on the opposite page to create your own food journal. Or to purchase the same food journal that the Biggest Losers use, go to www.biggestloser.com.

Faithfully keeping a calorie budget and a food journal will allow you to see in black and white the foods and habits that are helping you reach your goals and that are hindering your efforts. Exploring new food and recipe possibilities is one key to mastering this approach. Another important tactic is learning how to spot the foods that overstimulate your appetite and lead to uncontrolled eating.

Season 11's Jen Jacobs says that closely tracking her calories allowed her to make an easy swap

Sample Food Journal Page

	Calories	Carbohydrate (45%)	Protein (30%)	Fat (25%)
Sample Goal	1,200	540	360	300

Meal/ Time	Food	Calories	Carbohydrate	Protein	Fat
	Totals				
	Goal Totals				
	+/-				

and save a handful of calories every day. "I've been putting unsweetened coconut milk on my cereal," she says. "It's tasty and delicious, and gives me enough energy to head up to the gym and get through a workout. It has less calories per serving than skim milk."

As you learn which foods work best for you, be sure to keep those foods on hand. Stock up on them at home, and whenever possible take them with you on the road. Similarly, try to keep trigger foods out of your home environment and avoid impulse eating when you're away from home.

Keeping a food journal is paramount to your successful weight-loss efforts. It will help you to not only track your daily calories, but also learn from your eating patterns. Be sure to keep a journal with you at all times so you can jot down the foods you eat throughout the day. (If you wait until the end of the day to write down everything, you're likely to forget some of the calories you consumed.) And remember—every bite, taste, and nibble counts! Season 12's Bonnie Griffin agrees that writing down every last bite was essential to her success. "Never guesstimate what you're eating," she advises. "If it's not written down, your food intake can really add up."

Weighing and Measuring

In order to accurately record the foods you eat in your food journal, you'll need to know a little bit about serving sizes. It's important to weigh and measure your food so that you'll know exactly how many calories it contains. It's useful to have the following tools (many of which you may already own) to help you measure your portion sizes:

- Liquid measuring cup (2-cup capacity)
- Set of dry measuring cups (includes 1 cup, ½ cup, ⅓ cup, and ¼ cup)
- Measuring spoons (includes 1 tablespoon, 1 teaspoon, ½ teaspoon, and ¼ teaspoon)
- The *Biggest Loser* food scale
- Calculator

Be sure that your food scale measures in grams (a gram is about $\frac{1}{28}$ of an ounce). Most of your weight measurements will be in ounces, but certain foods, such as nuts, are very concentrated in calories, so you may need to measure your portion size in grams. You can also rely on *The Biggest Loser Calorie Counter* to help you calculate calories when you're not in your kitchen.

For common measurements and conversions, refer to the "Conversion Table for Measuring Portion Sizes" on the opposite page. It will be essential as you try out new recipes and determine portion sizes for your food journal. When you're making your meals at home, be sure to weigh and measure your food after cooking. A food's weight can change dramatically once it has been cooked.

CONVERSION TABLE FOR MEASURING PORTION SIZES

Teaspoons	Tablespoons	Cups	Pints, quarts, gallons	Fluid ounces	Milliliters
¼ teaspoon					1 ml
½ teaspoon					2 ml
1 teaspoon	⅓ tablespoon				5 ml
3 teaspoons	1 tablespoon	1/16 cup		½ oz	15 ml
6 teaspoons	2 tablespoons	⅛ cup		1 oz	30 ml
12 teaspoons	4 tablespoons	¼ cup		2 oz	60 ml
16 teaspoons	5⅓ tablespoons	⅓ cup		2½ oz	75 ml
24 teaspoons	8 tablespoons	½ cup		4 oz	125 ml
32 teaspoons	10⅔ tablespoons	⅔ cup		5 oz	150 ml
36 teaspoons	12 tablespoons	¾ cup		6 oz	175 ml
48 teaspoons	16 tablespoons	1 cup	½ pint	8 oz	237 ml
		2 cups	1 pint	16 oz	473 ml
		3 cups		24 oz	710 ml
		4 cups	1 quart	32 oz	946 ml
		8 cups	½ gallon	64 oz	
		16 cups	1 gallon	128 oz	

For example, a boneless chicken breast that weighs about 4 ounces when raw will weigh about 3 ounces after cooking, but will contain the same number of calories. The same holds true for vegetables and some other foods. Dry cereals or grains, on the other hand, can double or even triple in volume after being cooked with water. Remember that an ounce of weight is not the same as a fluid ounce. You cannot convert the two without knowing the density of the ingredient you are measuring.

After measuring out your foods for a week or so, you'll be able to make fairly accurate estimates on your own. Over time, you'll know what an appropriate portion size looks like, whether you're making a meal at home or dining out. But when you first begin your weight-loss plan, these tools will help you get it just right.

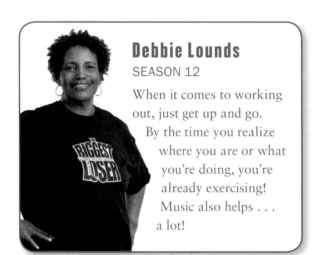

Debbie Lounds
SEASON 12

When it comes to working out, just get up and go. By the time you realize where you are or what you're doing, you're already exercising! Music also helps . . . a lot!

The Biggest Loser Plan

The *Biggest Loser* nutrition pyramid is made up of fruits and vegetables at its base, protein foods on the second tier, and whole grains on the third tier. The top tier is a 200-calorie budget for healthy fats and "extras."

On *The Biggest Loser* 4-3-2-1 plan, you will eat a daily minimum of 4 servings of fruits and vegetables, up to 3 servings of healthy protein, up to 2 servings of whole grains, and up to 1 serving of "extras."

45 Percent of Your Daily Calories: Vegetables, Fruits, and Whole Grains

At the base of the pyramid, fruits and vegetables supply most of your daily nutrients in the form of vitamins, minerals, and fiber, and contain relatively low numbers of calories. Aim for a minimum of 4 cups daily of a variety of fruits and nonstarchy vegetables. You can eat more than 4 servings a day of most fruits and vegetables if you wish, though the majority of your choices should be vegetables.

Vegetables: Serving size = 1 cup or 8 ounces

Tips for eating vegetables:

- When cooking vegetables, avoid added fat. Steam, grill, or stir-fry veggies in a nonstick pan with a spray (not a splash) of healthy oil.

THE 4-3-2-1 BIGGEST LOSER PYRAMID

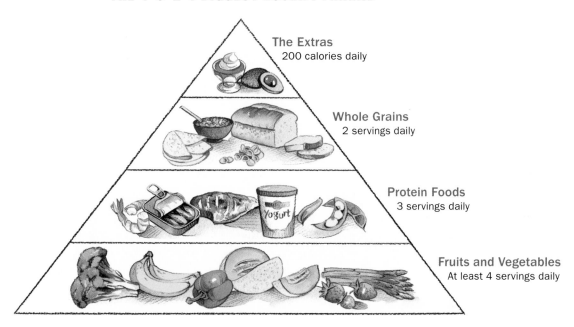

The Extras
200 calories daily

Whole Grains
2 servings daily

Protein Foods
3 servings daily

Fruits and Vegetables
At least 4 servings daily

- Try to eat at least one raw vegetable each day.

- Try a new vegetable each week so that you don't get bored with the same veggies.

- Eat a vegetable salad for lunch or dinner most days of the week.

- Keep precut vegetables such as bell peppers, celery, broccoli, and jicama in your fridge for easy snacking at home or to take to work or school.

- Starchier vegetables such as pumpkin, winter squash, and sweet potatoes are higher in calories and carbs, so limit them to one or two servings per week.

- Fresh vegetables are best, but you can choose frozen, as well. If you opt for canned, be sure to rinse the contents before eating, to wash away added salt.

Fruit: Serving size = 1 cup, 1 medium piece, or 8 ounces

Tips for eating fruit:

- Enjoy at least one whole fruit each day. Apples, oranges, pears, bananas, and grapes are all easily portable and can be eaten for snacks on the go.

- Dark green, light green, orange, purple, red, and yellow—savor fruits from different color groups. This ensures you're getting a variety of nutrients.

- Eat fruit for dessert! Many *Biggest Losers* who have a sweet tooth use this strategy.

- Opt for fresh fruit over dried fruits, which are more concentrated in calories and sugar and are less filling.

- Choose whole fruit rather than fruit juices. Fruit juice contains less fiber, so it's not as filling as whole fruit, and it's more concentrated in sugars, so it will cause a spike in your blood sugar. When you do choose juice, keep in mind that a serving size is 4 ounces (½ cup).

- Fresh fruit is preferable, but frozen fruit is fine as long as it's not packaged with added sugar or syrup. If you choose canned fruit, be sure it's packed in water.

Whole Grains: Serving size = 1 cup of cooked grains or 2 slices of bread

Choose whole grain foods in moderation, and select those with high fiber content. On *The Biggest Loser* plan, you will eat 2 servings of whole grains daily. When grains are refined, important nutrients are removed. All that's usually left is starch, which is loaded with carbohydrate calories and little else. Whole grains undergo minimal processing and thus retain most of their nutritional value. The whole grain family includes barley, corn, oats, quinoa, rice, and wheat. These are all great sources of protein, B vitamins, antioxidants, and fiber.

Tips for eating whole grains:

- When choosing bread products, read the label carefully. If it says "enriched," the product probably contains white flour—meaning it's low in fiber and nutrition.

- Choose breads with at least 2 grams of fiber per serving, but aim for 5 grams. When you read the ingredient list, look for "whole wheat" or "whole grain" among the first few ingredients. "Wheat flour" isn't necessarily whole wheat.

- Most packaged breakfast cereals are highly processed and loaded with added sugar. Choose

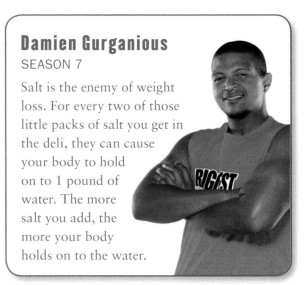

Damien Gurganious
SEASON 7

Salt is the enemy of weight loss. For every two of those little packs of salt you get in the deli, they can cause your body to hold on to 1 pound of water. The more salt you add, the more your body holds on to the water.

cereals with fewer than 5 grams of sugar and at least 5 grams of fiber per serving.

- White flour, white sugar, white bread, and packaged baked goods affect your blood sugar and insulin too quickly. You don't want an excess of either in your bloodstream. Unlike their whole grain counterparts, these foods also lack antioxidants and fiber. Choose whole grains, which will keep you feeling fuller longer.

30 Percent of Your Daily Calories: Protein

Protein is a macronutrient found in meat, fish, eggs, poultry, and dairy products, and in smaller amounts in beans, nuts, and whole grains. Protein is required to build and repair muscle, skin, hair, blood vessels, and other bodily tissues. Generally speaking, any food containing at least 9 grams of protein per serving is a high-protein food.

Lean proteins contain valuable nutrients that can help you achieve a healthy weight. Include protein with each meal and each snack so your body can benefit from it all day long. When you haven't eaten enough protein, you might find yourself running low on energy or suffering from muscle fatigue. Try to eat a little bit of protein or drink a protein shake within 30 minutes after a workout to help your muscles repair. In addition to helping build muscle, protein also promotes the feeling of satiety, or fullness, thus curbing your appetite and

keeping you from consuming extra calories. When combined with a carbohydrate (such as a piece of fruit), protein helps slow the release of blood sugar, sustaining your energy for longer periods of time.

Choose a variety of proteins to make up your 3 daily servings. Try to limit consumption of lean red meat to twice a week and avoid processed meats, such as bologna, hot dogs, and sausage, which are typically high in sodium and contain nitrates. Fish is an excellent source of protein, omega-3 fatty acids, vitamin E, and selenium.

To figure out how many grams of protein should constitute each of your 3 daily servings, use the formula below, which uses an 1,800-calorie budget as an example.

1,800 × 0.30 = 540 calories from protein

Then convert the calories to grams.

540 / 4 calories per gram = 135 grams of protein

You can then allocate protein goals for each meal and snack, based on your total daily protein intake. Daily protein servings, using the example above, might look like this:

Breakfast: 33 grams

Snack 1: 17 grams

Lunch: 34 grams

Snack 2: 17 grams

Dinner: 34 grams

Animal Protein: Serving size = 1 cup or 8 ounces

Meat

Choose lean cuts of meat, such as pork tenderloin and beef round, chuck, sirloin, or tenderloin. USDA Choice or USDA Select grades of beef usually have lower fat content. Avoid meat that is heavily marbled and remove any visible fat. Try to find ground meat that is at least 95 percent lean.

Poultry

The leanest poultry is the skinless white meat from the breast of chicken or turkey. When purchasing ground chicken or turkey, ask for the white meat.

Seafood

Seafood is an excellent source of protein, omega-3 fatty acids, vitamin E, and selenium. When you're buying seafood, go for options that are rich in omega-3 fatty acids, such as herring, mackerel, salmon, sardines (water packed), trout, and tuna.

Dairy: Serving size = 1 cup or 8 ounces

Top choices include fat-free milk, 1 percent (low-fat) milk, buttermilk, plain fat-free or low-fat yogurt, fat-free or low-fat yogurt with fruit (no sugar added), fat-free or low-fat cottage cheese, and fat-free or low-fat ricotta cheese. Light soy milks and soy yogurts are also fine, but if you eat soy because of a dairy intolerance or allergy, be sure to select soy products that are fortified with calcium. Egg whites are another excellent source of fat-free protein.

If you're not eating 3 servings of dairy per day, *The Biggest Loser* nutrition team recommends that you consider taking a calcium supplement.

Vegetarian Protein: Serving size = 1 cup or 8 ounces

Good sources of vegetarian protein include beans, nuts and seeds, and traditional soy foods, such as tofu and edamame. Many of these foods are also loaded with fiber.

25 Percent of Your Daily Calories: Good Fats

Healthy fats play a role in weight loss because they help you feel full and satisfied. But remember: Even good fats are a concentrated source of calories, and as such, you need to monitor your serving sizes carefully. Many of your fat calories will be hidden in your carbohydrate and protein food choices. You will have a small budget of leftover calories to spend on healthy fat and "extras."

Fats should make up no more than 25 percent of your total daily calories, and saturated fats should account for no more than 10 percent of your daily calorie budget. Here's how to calculate your daily fat intake, again based on the example of an 1,800-calorie budget.

Multiply your total daily calorie budget by 0.25 to see how many calories can come from fat.

$$1,800 \times 0.25 = 450$$

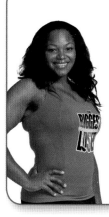

Andrea Hough
SEASON 9

Here's my new favorite snack. Cut an apple into slices. Then take some nonfat Greek yogurt, add a few chopped walnuts, and sprinkle a little natural sweetener like Truvía over it. It tastes like apple pie!

So with an 1,800-calorie budget, up to 450 of the daily calories may come from fat.

One gram of fat contains 9 calories. So divide the number of calories from fat that you're allotted each day (in this case, 450) by 9.

$$450 / 9 = 50$$

A person with an 1,800-calorie budget would consume no more than 50 grams of fat daily.

Healthy Fats

- Choose olive oil, canola oil, flaxseed oil, or walnut oil for salads, cooking, and baking.
- When adding fat to a sandwich, try using reduced-fat mayonnaise or a little mashed-up avocado.
- Snack on nuts and seeds in moderation. Nut butters, trail mix, and raw nuts pack a powerful energy punch and supply a good dose of unsaturated fat. Keep portion sizes moderate; for example, 14 walnut halves make a 1-ounce serving.
- Choose unsaturated fats. Many unsaturated fats, classified as monounsaturated or polyunsaturated, can lower your LDL (bad) cholesterol and raise your HDL (good) cholesterol.
- Avoid trans fats, an artificial fat found in hard margarines and vegetable shortenings, packaged baked goods, and foods fried in hydrogenated fat. Carefully read labels of packaged foods. If you see the words *hydrogenated* or *partially hydrogenated,* put the package back on the shelf.

Decoding Food Packaging

Keeping a food journal will require you to become an expert at reading food labels and Nutrition Facts panels. When you're shopping for healthy foods, labels can help you choose between similar products based on calorie and nutrient (such as fat, protein, or fiber) content.

On page 18 you'll find an example of a typical food label. It contains a lot of information, but here are the essential facts you need to know in order to make healthy choices.

Serving size: Everything else on the label (calories, grams of fat, etc.) is based on this measurement.

Just because a food label suggests a certain portion doesn't mean that it's the right serving size for you. Look at the calorie and fat content that corresponds to the serving size. If you need to, cut the serving size in half.

Calories: This lists calories per serving. Be sure that the number of calories you record in your food journal reflects the number of calories you've eaten. If the label indicates that a serving is 1 cup and you ate 2 cups, you need to double the calories that you record in your journal to match your double serving.

Total fat: The number of fat grams in a product reflects the sum of three kinds of fat: saturated fat, polyunsaturated fat, and monounsaturated fat. Pay special attention to the numbers of calories in "light," reduced-fat, low-fat, and fat-free products. When the fat is removed from many recipes, salt or sugar is sometimes added to enhance the flavor.

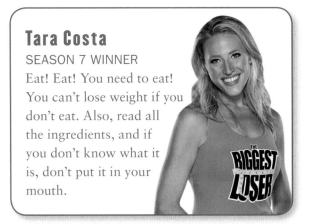

Tara Costa

SEASON 7 WINNER

Eat! Eat! You need to eat! You can't lose weight if you don't eat. Also, read all the ingredients, and if you don't know what it is, don't put it in your mouth.

Nutrition Facts

Serving Size
Servings Per Container

Amount Per Serving	
Calories 0	Calories from Fat 0

	% Daily Value*
Total Fat 0g	0%
Saturated Fat 0g	0%
Trans Fat 0g	
Cholesterol 0mg	0%
Sodium 0mg	0%
Total Carbohydrate 0g	0%
Dietary Fiber 0g	0%
Soluble Fiber 0g	0%
Insoluble Fiber 0g	0%
Sugars 0g	
Protein 0g	

Vitamin A 0%	•	Vitamin C 0%	
Calcium 0%	•	Iron 0%	
Phosphorus 0%	•	Magnesium 0%	

* Percent Daily Values are based on a 2,000 calo-rie diet. Your daily values may be higher or lower depending on your calorie needs:

		Calories:	2,000	2,500
Total Fat	Less than		0g	0g
Sat Fat	Less than		0g	0g
Cholesterol	Less than		0mg	0mg
Sodium	Less than		0mg	0mg
Potassium			0mg	0mg
Total Carbohydrate			0g	0g
Dietary Fiber			0g	0g

Calories per gram:
Fat 0 • Carbohydrate 0 • Protein 0

This can result in a fat-free or low-fat product that actually contains more calories than the regular version.

Saturated fat: Less than one-third of your daily fat grams should come from saturated fats, which are derived mainly from animal products and are solid at room temperature (such as butter and shortening). Some plant oils, such as coconut oil and palm oil, also contain saturated fats. The saturated fat from animal foods is the primary source of cholesterol.

Sodium: For most people, the daily recommended sodium intake is no more than 2,400 milligrams. Some of the foods you eat each day will have more, others less. Aim for an average of no more than 240 milligrams of sodium in each meal or snack.

Total carbohydrate: This number is calculated by adding grams of complex carbohydrates plus grams of fiber plus grams of sugar. If the total carbohydrate number is more than double the amount of sugar, that means there are more "good carbs" than "bad carbs" in the food.

Dietary fiber: Fiber is found in plant foods but not in animal foods. Unless you're on a fiber-restricted diet, aim to consume at least 25 to 35 grams of fiber per day.

Sugar: The sugars in a food can be naturally occurring or added. Check the ingredient list to find out and avoid eating foods that contain processed sugar, such as high-fructose corn syrup. The total grams of carbohydrates in a food serving should be more than twice the number of grams of sugar.

Protein: If a food has more than 9 grams of protein per serving, it's considered a high-protein food. It's important to eat foods that are high in protein when you're trying to lose weight, because protein is a great source of energy and helps you feel full.

Ingredient List

A product's ingredients are listed in order of decreasing weight. If the first few ingredients listed include any form of sugar (cane sugar, corn syrup, sucrose, and so on) or fats and oils, the food is probably not a good choice for weight loss. Also, look for products with a short list of ingredients that you recognize. A long list of strange-sounding ingredients is always a red flag. Leave those products on the shelf at the grocery store—don't put them on the shelf of your pantry.

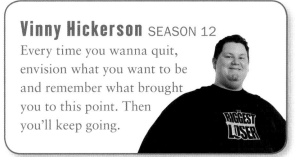

Vinny Hickerson SEASON 12
Every time you wanna quit, envision what you want to be and remember what brought you to this point. Then you'll keep going.

No Excuses Fitness

As you know by now, weight loss is all about calories in and calories out. Calculating a calorie budget, planning your meals and snacks, and tracking what you eat in a food journal are all great ways to make sure you are taking in the right number and right kind of calories. But what about the "calories out" part of the equation?

The contestants at the Ranch put in long, hard workouts every day. But you don't have to work out for hours with Bob and Jillian to see results. If you're not already active, start incorporating more activity into your day. Walk or bike instead of driving, take the stairs instead of the elevator, or treat your dog to an extra-long walk. It doesn't matter how small you start. You just have to get moving.

If you already exercise moderately, consider increasing the duration (the amount of time you exercise) and the intensity (how hard you exercise) to see more results. If you typically walk or run on a treadmill for 30 minutes, try adding an incline, holding some hand weights, or increasing your time by 10 minutes. If you take a beginner's yoga class once a week, ask yourself if you're ready to move to the intermediate level or take the class twice a week. The more you put into your fitness regimen, the more you will get out of it.

Here are some tools to help you get moving, no matter what your fitness level is today.

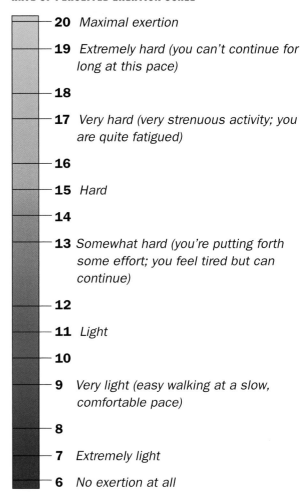

RATE OF PERCEIVED EXERTION SCALE

- **20** *Maximal exertion*
- **19** *Extremely hard (you can't continue for long at this pace)*
- **18**
- **17** *Very hard (very strenuous activity; you are quite fatigued)*
- **16**
- **15** *Hard*
- **14**
- **13** *Somewhat hard (you're putting forth some effort; you feel tired but can continue)*
- **12**
- **11** *Light*
- **10**
- **9** *Very light (easy walking at a slow, comfortable pace)*
- **8**
- **7** *Extremely light*
- **6** *No exertion at all*

Make a Plan

Studies show that people who plan ahead for their workouts are generally more successful than those who wing it. Decide when you want to work out and put it in your day planner. Log that time as yours. After you've exercised, record your accomplishments in this journal.

- Set an alarm as a reminder to work out. Or schedule a reminder on your computer, if that's where you spend most of your day.
- Pack your gym bag the night before so that you can grab it and go in the morning.

Build a Team

At the Ranch, contestants are divided into teams to provide support and guidance for one another. You'll need that encouragement, too!

- Plan walking activities with your kids or encourage a friend to become an exercise buddy.
- Look for workout partners online through sites like www.biggestloserclub.com or through your local colleges, churches, and community centers.

Be Consistent

Experts suggest that it takes 21 days of consistent behavior to form a habit, so don't get discouraged after only a couple of days. Find small ways to stay active, and before you know it, your body will start to crave exercise.

Get FITTE

FITTE is a quick, handy acronym to help you remember all the elements of an exercise routine that you need to improve your fitness. It's a good way, especially for beginners, to start thinking about working out. As you begin to make exercise a part of your lifestyle, you'll want to vary or increase some or all elements of the FITTE principle:

Frequency: How often you work out

Intensity: How hard you work out (measuring with a heart rate monitor or using rate of perceived exertion)

Time: The duration of your workout

Type: The kind of exercise you're doing

Enjoyment: How much pleasure you get out of the activity

Frequency

The American Council on Exercise recommends 20 to 30 minutes of cardiovascular exercise 3 to 5 days a week (depending on intensity; a shorter workout duration calls for more intensity) and strength training at least twice a week. You can combine cardio and strength on some days or keep them separate.

Intensity: Load, Speed, and Effort

There are many ways to increase or decrease intensity.

- Load: This is the amount of resistance you use in your workout. For strength training, you can use your own body weight as resistance or increase the load (and intensity) by adding weights.

- **Speed:** During your cardio workouts, you can amp up intensity by simply going faster. It will help you burn more calories and strengthen your heart. You can vary speed in the strength exercises, too. When exercising with dumbbells, keep your speed under control to ensure that you never swing the weights.

- **Effort:** This is one of the most common ways to vary intensity. The Rate of Perceived Exertion (RPE), shown on page 20, is an easy-to-follow self-measurement. Use the rating scale to gauge how your body feels when you're working out. RPE ranges from 6 (no exertion at all) to 20 (maximal exertion).

Calculating Your Target Heart Rate

The rate of perceived exertion scale relates to your exercise heart rate as well. We all have a resting heart rate (our pulse rate when we are immobile), a maximum heart rate (the highest rate we should reach in a workout), and a target heart rate zone (for maximum fat burning). Your target heart rate—the rate that you should aim to achieve in your workouts—can be easily calculated, once you know your maximum heart rate. To find your maximum heart rate, follow this simple formula:

220 – your age = Maximum heart rate

So, for a 35-year-old, the maximum heart rate is 185 (220 – 35 = 185).

Now, to find your target heart rate zone, you're going to use the number you just calculated for your maximum heart rate:

**Low-range target heart rate =
Maximum heart rate × 0.80**

**High-range target heart rate =
Maximum heart rate × 0.85**

So, for the same 35-year-old:

- The target heart rate (low range) would be 148 (185 × 80% = 148).

- The target heart rate (high range) would be 157 (185 × 85% = 157).

This person should aim to keep his or her heart rate between 148 and 157 when exercising.

Studies have shown a correlation between rate of perceived exertion and heart rate, with heart rate equaling about 10 times the RPE you've reached. For example, if you're working out at an 11 on the scale, your heart rate should be approximately 110. For the 35-year-old, this would not be

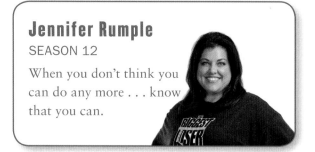

Jennifer Rumple
SEASON 12

When you don't think you can do any more . . . know that you can.

in the target heart rate zone. That person would need to increase the intensity and be more in the 14 to 16 range to achieve the 148 to 157 target heart rate zone. Looking at the RPE scale, this makes sense, as that range represents "somewhat hard" to "hard."

Time

Time (or duration) is how long you actually exercise. We're all challenged to find time to exercise, but it's important to stick to your exercise schedule and put in as many minutes or hours as you can dedicate if you want to achieve your weight-loss goals.

Type

The type of exercise you choose will have a great impact on whether you can maintain a fitness program. If you prefer, fulfill your 30 minutes of aerobic exercise with cycling rather than walking. Studies show that you'll be more likely to stick to an exercise program if you like what you're doing. Other options are swimming, jumping rope, and aerobics classes. If you don't enjoy lifting dumbbells, try using tubing, elastic bands, medicine balls, weighted water balls, and stability balls (go to www.biggestloser.com for products).

Enjoyment

You'll find former *Biggest Loser* contestants training for marathons, competing in triathlons and Ironmans, teaching yoga classes, rock climbing—and doing just about any other type of physical activity you can imagine. Once you find a form of exercise you love and look forward to doing, you're more likely to stick to your workout schedule and meet your goals. Many of the contestants who once professed to "hate" exercising find that it's something they simply can't live without today. Ali Vincent, a self-proclaimed exercise addict, says she can hardly believe that she used to sit around and watch TV at night. "I just don't feel right if I don't go to the gym," she says. "It's not just something I have to do, it's something I want to do."

In the pages that follow, you'll discover that it only requires 20 minutes a day to start burning more calories and get one step closer to your weight-loss goals. So get ready, get set . . . no more excuses! You have the time to get fit and healthy—20 minutes a day is a worthy investment in your future. As *Biggest Loser* trainer Dolvett Quince would say, it's time to "change your life, one rep at a time."

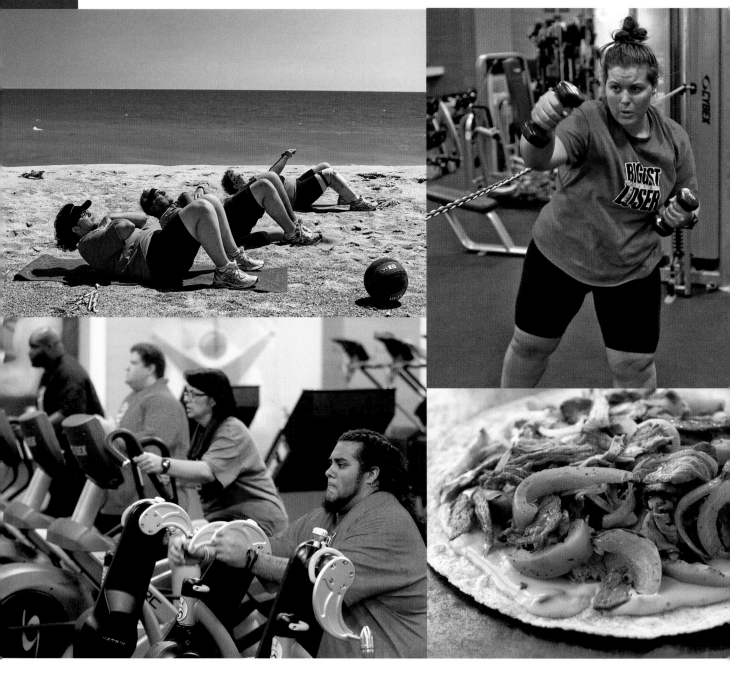

20 Minutes to a Better Body

Whether you have 10 pounds or 100 to lose, when you think about reaching your goal weight, the idea of hitting your target can feel overwhelming. Just as you need to break down your eating into manageable increments—setting a calorie budget and approaching it day by day, meal by meal—the same principle should be applied to your fitness routine.

The Centers for Disease Control and Prevention (CDC) recommends that everyone, regardless of weight-loss goals, should aim for 150 minutes of moderate cardiovascular exercise, or 75 minutes of vigorous exercise plus two strength training sessions weekly. You can combine cardio and strength training on some days or keep them separate. The most important thing is that you get active. As Season 12 contestant Jessica Limpert puts it, "If you're not moving, you're not losing!"

In the 20 minutes it takes you to flip channels, talk to a friend on the phone, or drive to the mall, you can squeeze in a 20-minute workout. In the pages that follow, you'll find six 20-minute circuits geared toward specific fitness levels. It's important to note that anyone who is new to a fitness program should consult a doctor before exercising. And as always, drink plenty of fluids to stay hydrated.

Biggest Loser trainer Bob Harper suggests keeping a daily or weekly workout log to help you stay on track. "It's a great strategy to make sure you're progressing properly," he advises. "Be sure to note the frequency, intensity, and duration of your workout. Watching your improvement is a great motivator, and writing it down will help you stay on track."

Before you begin any of these 20-minute workouts, warm up for 5 minutes with any basic movement—

such as walking, marching in place, or doing alternating knee lifts—to elevate your heart rate slightly and raise your body temperature. To add intensity and increase calorie burn, perform each of the exercises in a circuit, with little to no rest between sets. Follow each workout with a light stretch for the major muscle groups.

So let's get started. You're just 20 minutes away from getting closer to your goal weight!

20-Minute Fitness for Beginners: Workout 1

Cardio

Walk at a brisk pace for 10 minutes. You can do this on a treadmill at home, at the gym, or simply by walking around your neighborhood.

Mobility and Strength Training

Perform each of the exercises on the pages that follow for 1 minute, moving through the circuit. When you've finished the circuit, repeat it, for a total of 10 minutes of mobility and strength training.

MAKE A DIFFERENCE IN 20 MINUTES

Scrub Your Way Thin

Sure, cleaning the house is a drag, and many people like to pawn off the hardest chores on their unsuspecting spouses. But before you ask your hubby to cut the grass or your wife to do the windows, consider that 20 minutes of vigorous cleaning can burn up to 80 calories. So take back the reins of the vacuum and clean your way to calorie burn!

SHOULDER ROLL

Stand with your feet shoulder-width apart. Keep your arms at your sides and your abdominal muscles engaged. Roll your shoulders forward in a circle for 15 seconds. Then roll your shoulders backward for 15 seconds. Repeat forward and back for a total of 1 minute.

Tips

- As you roll your shoulders, try to make each circle a little bigger than the previous one. Think of lifting your shoulders all the way up to your ears, then pulling your shoulder blades together, then pushing your shoulder blades to the floor, and finally opening your back as you pull the front of your shoulders forward.

- Don't allow your lower back or your hips to move.

- Keep your neck neutral and your head still.

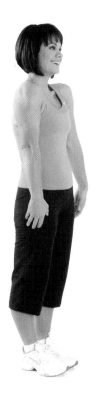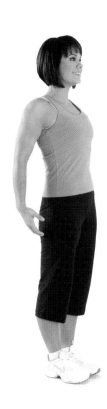

SIDE BEND

Stand with your feet shoulder-width apart and your arms by your sides. Inhale and extend your right arm toward the ceiling. As you exhale, bend at your waist to your left and extend your arm over your head and to the left. Inhale as you bring your body back up and exhale as you release your arm. Repeat with your left arm as you bend to the right. Repeat slowly, alternating sides, for 1 minute (about 4 repetitions on each side).

Tips

- Keep your weight evenly distributed on both feet, especially during the side bend.
- Think of reaching up and out, rather than down and collapsing into your side.
- Don't allow your lower back to arch or your knees to lock.

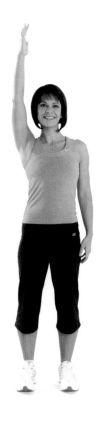
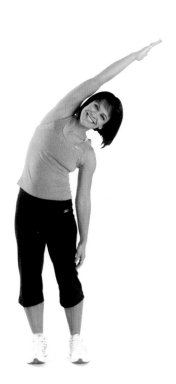

LOWER-BACK MOBILITY

Stand with your feet a little wider than shoulder-width apart. Hinge forward from the hips and place your hands on your thighs. Your back should be neutral, and your shoulders should be away from your ears. Inhale to prepare, and as you exhale, tuck your tailbone under and round your back, pulling your tailbone up toward the ceiling. Inhale and reverse the movement by arching your back, tilting your tailbone up toward the ceiling. Repeat slowly for 1 minute (about 12 to 16 repetitions).

Tips

- Start the movement with your breath.
- Keep your abdominal muscles tight during the back arch. Don't allow your belly to relax.
- Think of drawing a semicircle with your tailbone.

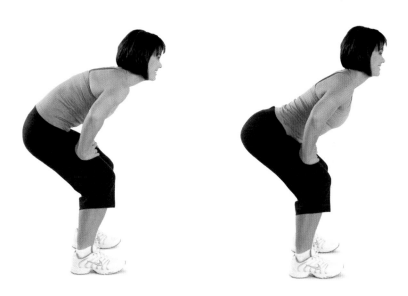

DYNAMIC LATERAL LUNGE

Stand with your feet fairly wide, your shoulders rolled back, and your abdominal muscles engaged. Bend your left knee and shift your weight to your left leg, placing your hands on your left thigh for support. Allow your torso to move slightly forward, but keep your left knee behind your toes. Press into the floor, straighten your left leg, and return to the starting position. Repeat to the right. Alternate right and left for 1 minute (about 6 repetitions on each side).

Tips

- Don't let your back round as you sit back into your hips. Keep your head up and your shoulders rolled back and down.

- Keep the opposite leg straight to feel the inner thigh lengthen.

- As you come back to the standing position, squeeze your buttocks to bring your pelvis upright.

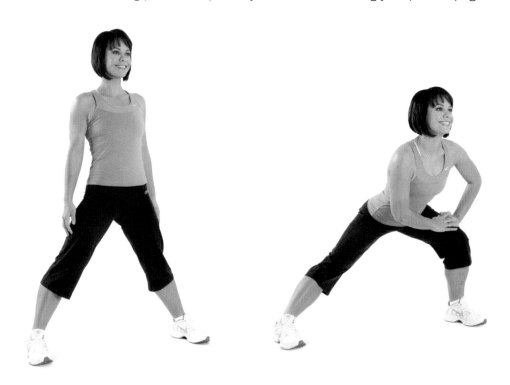

TORSO ROTATION

Stand with your feet slightly wider than your hips, shoulders rolled back, and your abdominal muscles engaged. Bring your arms in front of your body, cross them, and grab your elbows, arms parallel to the floor. Bend your knees slightly and lengthen your spine toward the ceiling. Keeping your hips where they are, rotate your torso to the left. Return to center and repeat to the right. Continue alternating sides for 1 minute (about 12 to 16 repetitions).

Tips

- As you rotate to the left, think of pressing your left hip forward to keep your hips stable.

- Lift as you rotate to avoid "grinding" into your lower back.

- Aim to keep your arms in front of your chest.

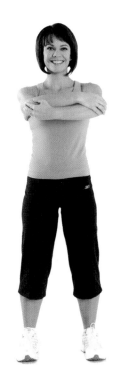 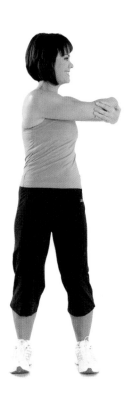

20-Minute Fitness for Beginners: Workout 2

Cardio

Climb the stairs on a stair machine at the gym, or simply walk up and down the stairs in your own home at a brisk pace for 10 minutes.

Mobility and Strength Training

If you have an exercise mat or yoga mat, lay it on the floor. If not, find a carpeted area for the next 10 minutes of your workout. You can perform the following exercises in socks or barefoot, but gym shoes are not needed. Be sure you have enough room around you to extend your arms behind your head.

As you perform the exercises that follow, concentrate on your breathing. Breathe in as you relax your muscles, and exhale slowly as you contract your muscles.

Perform each of these exercises for 1 minute, moving through the circuit. When you've finished the circuit, repeat it a second time, for a total of 10 minutes of mobility and strength training.

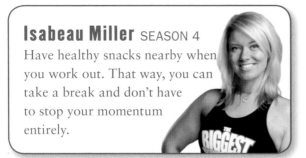

Isabeau Miller SEASON 4

Have healthy snacks nearby when you work out. That way, you can take a break and don't have to stop your momentum entirely.

SINGLE LEG STRETCH

Lie down on your back. Bend your knees and lift your legs and feet, so that your shins are parallel to the floor. Slowly curl your torso to lift your head and shoulders off the floor, keeping your spine flexed, engaging your core muscles, and placing your hands on your shins. Extend your left leg in front of you as far as you can while maintaining control and keeping your hips stable, placing your left hand on your right leg below the knee and your right hand on your right shin. Hold for several seconds then, maintaining a stable pelvis, switch legs and hands and hold again.

Tips

- Drop your shoulders down and back.
- Slow, controlled movements will help you keep your hips stable and avoid any rocking motion in your torso.

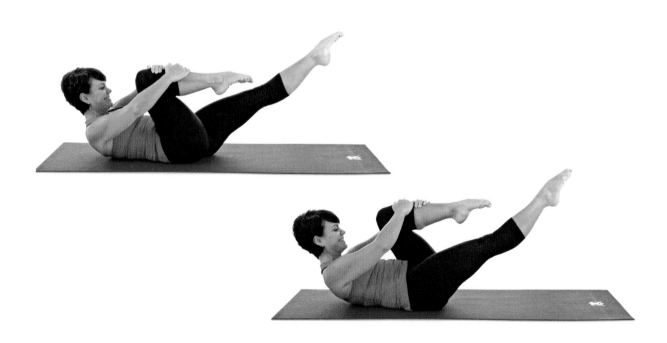

CRISSCROSS

Lie down on your back. Bend your knees and lift your legs and feet, so that your shins are parallel to the floor. Slowly curl your torso to lift your head and shoulders off the floor, keeping your spine flexed, engaging your core muscles, and placing your hands behind your head. Extend your left leg in front of you as far as you can while maintaining control and keeping your hips stable, and cross your left shoulder toward your right knee. Hold for 2 seconds. Then, maintaining a stable pelvis, switch legs and shoulders and hold again. Alternate right and left for 1 minute.

Tips

- Drop your shoulders down and back.
- Slow, controlled movements will help you keep your hips stable and avoid any rocking motion in your torso.
- Keep your chest open and draw the bottom of your rib cage to the opposite hip.

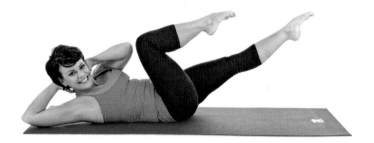

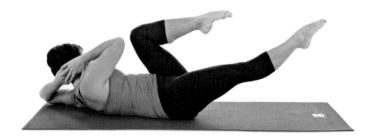

SWIMMING

Lie on your stomach with your legs and arms extended on the floor so that your body is in one long, straight line. Engage your abdominals and lift your arms and legs so that you extend your spine and hips. Begin a "swimming" flutter motion by lifting your right leg and left arm higher, then lowering them as you lift your left leg and right arm higher. Continue to alternate sides for 1 minute.

Tips

- To avoid compressing your lower back, imagine lengthening out as opposed to lifting up.
- Engage your core during this entire exercise.
- Drop your shoulders down and back, and keep your head in line with your spine.
- Avoid any rocking movement of your hips and torso.

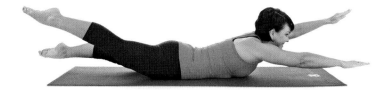

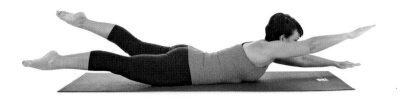

FRONT AND BACK

Lie down on your left side and form one line from the crown of your head to your hips, and extend your legs slightly forward. Rest your head on your left arm and place your right hand on the floor in front of you for support. Flex your foot and hip to bring your right leg forward. Pulse the leg upward two times, then point your foot and extend the same leg behind you. Do 8 to 10 repetitions, then roll over and exercise with your left leg, for about 1 minute total.

Tips

- Reach out through your heel when your leg is forward and reach through your toes when your leg is extended back.

- Keep your hips stacked during the entire range of motion; avoid any rocking or tilting of your pelvis.

- Don't allow your back to round or arch. The only movement should be in the raised leg and hip.

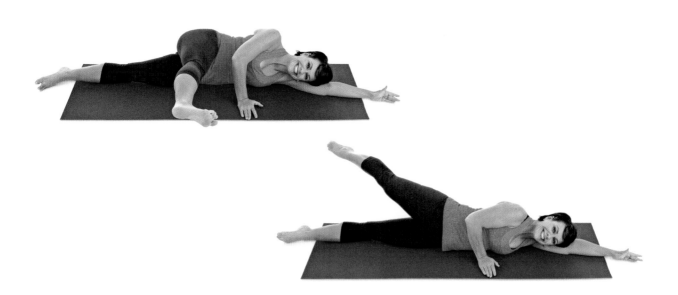

LEG PULLUP

Begin in a reverse plank position, hands on the floor behind you, palms pointing toward your feet. Facing the ceiling, support your weight on your hands and feet only, with your hips lifted, your hands under your shoulders, and your feet pointed. Tuck your chin, engage your core, and lift your right leg up toward the ceiling, keeping your hips lifted and shoulders pulled down and away from your ears. Hold for 2 seconds, then lower your leg. Repeat with your left leg. Continue alternating sides for 1 minute.

Tips

- As you lift your leg, avoid arching or rounding your back; keep your hips level.
- Keep your ribs "soft" and press your hands into the floor so that your shoulders stay down and away from your ears.
- Imagine your hips being suspended from the ceiling.
- If you need to make the move a little easier, lift your leg only a few inches off the floor.

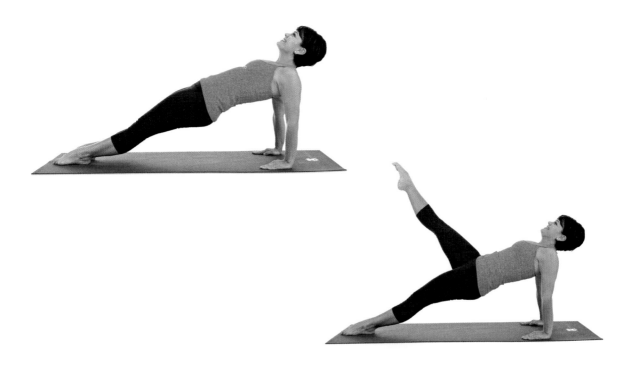

20-Minute Fitness for Intermediate Exercisers: Workout 1

Cardio

Jog or walk/jog for 10 minutes on a treadmill at home or at the gym, or simply walk/jog around your neighborhood.

Strength Training

The exercises that follow target your upper body. You will need an exercise band or tubing with handles to complete this circuit. If you don't have tubing, you can substitute dumbbells. Tubing is ideal, as it offers a different type of resistance (generally of less intensity) and makes it easier to transition between exercises.

Once you've completed one circuit of these five exercises, complete a second circuit, for a total of 10 minutes of strength training.

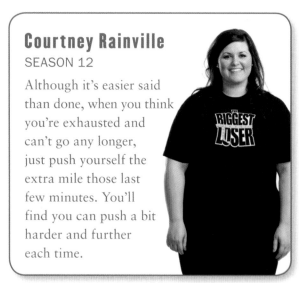

Courtney Rainville
SEASON 12

Although it's easier said than done, when you think you're exhausted and can't go any longer, just push yourself the extra mile those last few minutes. You'll find you can push a bit harder and further each time.

REAR FLY

Begin by holding the handles of the tubing in each hand. Step on the tubing with one foot and hinge forward from the hips with your knees slightly bent. Keeping your spine neutral and your abdominals engaged, pull the handles up and out to the sides of your body, squeezing the muscles in your upper back and mid-back. Hold for a moment, then release the tubing back down toward the floor. Repeat for 1 minute.

Tips

- Avoid rounding your back.

- Control the movement and don't allow your elbows to lock on the downward motion of the exercise.

- Keep your navel pulled in and your abdominals engaged at all times.

- Keep your arms in line with your shoulders as you pull the handles of the tubing up and out to the sides of your body. Don't allow your shoulders to hunch up to your ears.

FEEL THE BURN

To challenge your balance and engage your core and lower body even more, lift your back leg in a slow, controlled movement as you extend your arms.

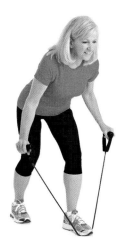
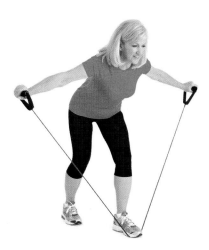

STATIONARY LUNGE

Begin in a staggered stance, with your left leg forward and your right leg back, heel off the floor. Place the tubing under your left foot, and hold the handles at your hips or shoulders. Keeping your spine neutral, your shoulders over your hips, and your abdominals engaged, bend both knees until your left thigh is parallel to the floor and your right knee is a few inches off the floor. Hold for a moment, then straighten both legs. Repeat on the other side. Continue alternating sides for 1 minute.

Tips

- Avoid rounding or arching your back.
- Keep your navel pulled in at all times.
- In the lunge, keep your left shin perpendicular to the floor so that your knee is directly over your ankle.
- Don't let your left knee move past your toes.

FEEL THE BURN

Choke up on the tubing to create additional resistance for more muscle burn. For even more of a challenge, raise your arms up higher into an overhead press as you lunge.

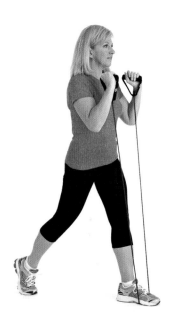
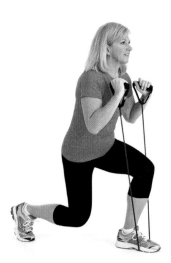

CHEST PRESS

Stand with your feet a little wider than hip-width apart. Take your tubing around your mid-back and grab the handles with each hand so that the tubing is under your armpits. If the tubing is too long, double it up so that both handles are in your right hand. Inhale deeply, and as you exhale, press both arms forward, keeping your chest lifted and your navel pulled toward your spine. Slowly bend your elbows and bring the tubing back toward your armpits. Repeat for 1 minute.

Tips

- Avoid arching your back or letting your chest cave in.
- Control the movement and don't allow your elbows to lock as you press out.
- Keep your navel pulled in at all times.
- Keep your wrists in line with your elbows and slightly below your shoulders.

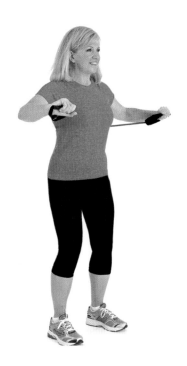 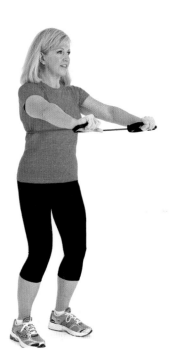

BICEPS CURL

Hold a dumbbell in each hand. Draw your navel to your spine, roll your shoulders back and down, and soften your knees. Slowly bend your elbows and bring the dumbbells up to your shoulders. Squeeze your biceps, then slowly return the dumbbells to the starting position. Repeat for 1 minute.

Tips

- Avoid arching your back or letting your chest cave in.
- Control the movement and don't allow your elbows to lock as you extend your arms.
- Keep your navel pulled in at all times.
- Keep your elbows slightly in front of your torso.

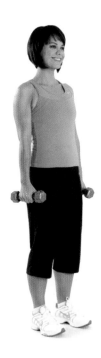 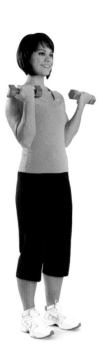

LATERAL RAISE

Hold a handle of the tubing in each hand. Step on the tubing in a narrow stance and hold the handles next to your thighs. Draw your navel to your spine, roll your shoulders back and down, and soften your knees. Slowly lift your arms out to the sides with your elbows slightly bent. Hold for a moment, relax your neck, and then slowly return the tubing to the starting position. Repeat for 1 minute.

Tips

- Avoid arching your back or letting your chest cave in.
- Control the movement and don't allow the tubing to pull your arms down.
- Keep your navel pulled in at all times.
- Keep your shoulders down and away from your ears, and hold your elbows slightly higher than your wrists.

FEEL THE BURN

To create more resistance and muscle burn, cross the handles of the tubing before you extend your arms out. To challenge your balance and engage your core and lower body, stand on one leg.

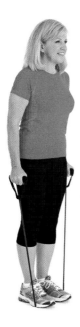
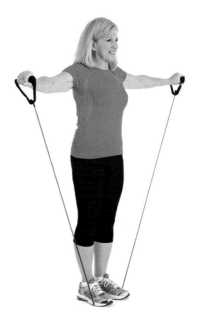

20-Minute Fitness for Intermediate Exercisers: Workout 2

Cardio

Ride a stationary bike for 10 minutes, either at the gym or at home, or simply hop on your bike and cycle a few quick laps around the block.

Strength Training

If you have an exercise mat or yoga mat, lay it on the floor. If not, find a carpeted area for the next 10 minutes of your workout. Be sure you have enough room around you to extend your arms behind your head.

All of the exercises in this circuit engage your core muscles. As you do each exercise, concentrate on breathing. Breathe in as you relax your muscles and exhale as you contract your muscles.

This circuit should take about 5 minutes to complete. When you've finished the first circuit, repeat it a second time, for a total of 10 minutes of strength training.

MAKE A DIFFERENCE IN 20 MINUTES

Take a Dip

The next time you're at the beach with your family, don't just watch your kids from the shoreline—dive in! Swimming is a huge calorie burner. Just 20 minutes of swimming with your kids can burn up to 135 calories—the equivalent of nine sugar-free popsicles.

PRESS-OUT

Lie on your back with your feet off the floor, knees bent at 90 degrees and shins parallel to the floor. With your hands by your sides, slowly extend one leg to a 45-degree diagonal, keeping your foot flexed. Hold for about 5 seconds, then bend your knee and return to the starting position. Switch legs and repeat. Continue, alternating legs, for a total of 12 repetitions with each leg, or 24 repetitions total.

Tips

- Keep your shoulders down and your upper torso still.
- Beginners can press the leg on a slight diagonal. Challengers should aim for the leg to be parallel to the floor.
- Keep breathing throughout the exercise.

FEEL THE BURN

Increase the intensity of your press-outs by extending your leg so that it is parallel to the floor and just a few inches above it, instead of at a 45-degree angle.

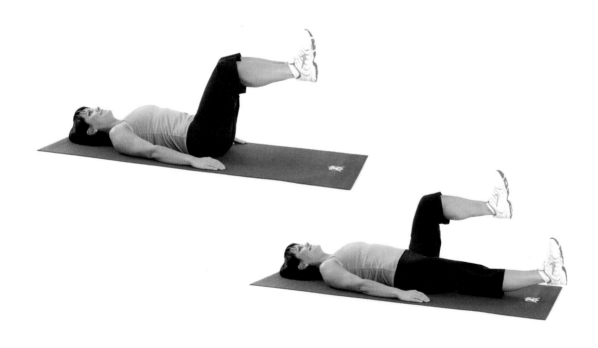

CRUNCH

Lie on your back with your knees bent, feet flat on the floor and toes pointing forward. Place your hands lightly behind your head, elbows bent. Engaging your core muscles, draw your navel toward your spine and slowly curl your head, neck, and shoulders off the floor toward your thighs. Pause at the top of the movement and squeeze your abs, then slowly lower back to the starting position. Continue for 1 minute, or about 12 to 15 repetitions.

Tips

- Come up off the floor only a few inches and keep your hips and lower back firmly pressed against the floor.

- Keep your head aligned with your spine and look past your knees.

- Try to release any tension in your neck and avoid pulling with your hands.

- Keep your core muscles engaged throughout the exercise.

FEEL THE BURN

To make your crunches more challenging, take your feet off the floor and bend your knees at a 90-degree angle so that your shins are parallel to the floor. Be careful to keep your hips firmly pressed to the floor as you do your crunches.

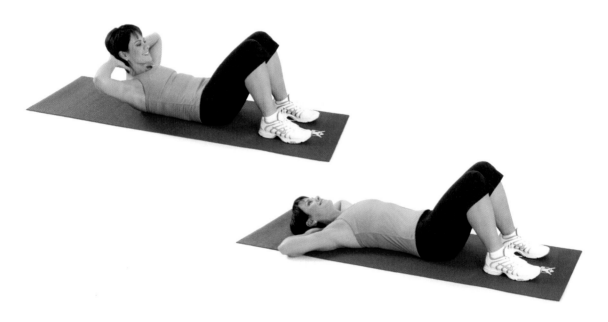

BICYCLE

Lie on your back with your feet off the floor, knees bent at a 90-degree angle and shins parallel to the floor. Place your hands lightly behind your head, elbows bent. Engaging your core muscles, draw your navel toward your spine and slowly move your right knee toward your left shoulder as you rotate your torso toward the knee. At the same time, extend your left leg outward. Pause for a moment and squeeze your abs, then switch sides. Continue alternating legs for 1 minute, or a total of about 15 to 20 repetitions.

Tips

- Keep your hips firmly planted on the floor to avoid rocking.
- Keep your elbows spread wide and avoid pulling on your neck.

FEEL THE BURN

To create a more intense workout, bring your lower leg parallel to the floor and, engaging your core, keep it just a few inches above the floor.

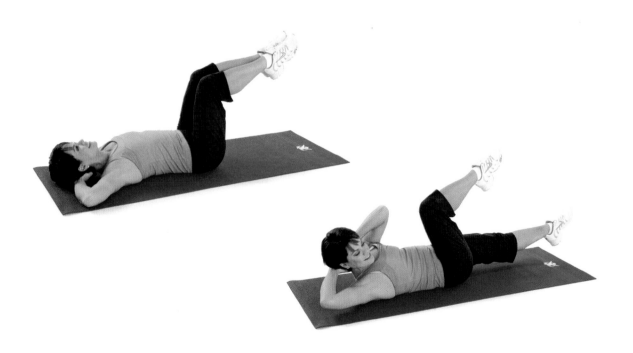

SUPERMAN

Lie facedown with your legs straight and your arms extended past your head. Gently contract the muscles in your lower back and mid-back to lift your torso off the floor, about 3 to 5 inches, while simultaneously lifting both legs off the floor—as if you're flying like Superman. Hold for several seconds, then return to the starting position. Continue for 1 minute, or about 12 to 15 repetitions.

Tips

- Think of reaching out and up with your spine, rather than up and back. This will take compression off your lumbar spine.

- Keep your shoulder blades down and back throughout the movement.

- Keep your breathing consistent throughout the movement.

FEEL THE BURN

Increase the burn by holding the Superman position for about 10 seconds and quickly paddling your legs, using small movements like you're swimming. Lower and return to starting position.

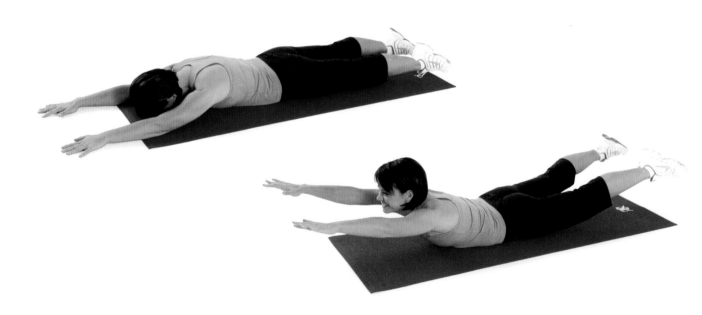

20-Minute Fitness for Advanced Exercisers: Workout 1 (All Cardio)

Run for 10 minutes on a treadmill at home or at the gym, or simply run around your neighborhood. For increased intensity, add speed work: Try running faster in two 1-minute bursts, one in the first 5 minutes of your run, and one in the last 5 minutes of your run.

JUMPING JACK

Begin with your feet together and your arms by your sides. Jump and spread your feet out to the sides about 2 to 2½ feet as you lift your arms to the side and over your head. Keep your knees soft and your core engaged as you land gently, with your heels on the floor. Immediately jump and pull your feet back in as you bring your arms to your sides. Repeat quickly for 2 minutes.

Tips

- Be sure to land gently, with your knees soft, to minimize impact on your spine and knees.
- Don't allow your knees to collapse inward. If you find your knees are doing this, don't jump out as wide.
- Keep your abdominals engaged and avoid arching your back.

FEEL THE BURN

To increase the intensity of your Jumping Jacks, try turning your torso left and right as you jump, and spread your feet wider.

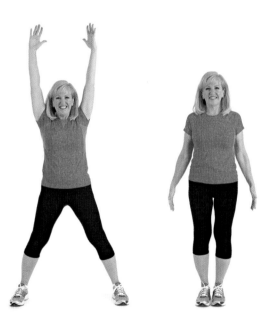

BURPEE

Stand with your feet at least hip-width apart and your arms by your sides. Squat down by bending your knees, keeping your back straight and your abs pulled in. Place your hands on the floor by your feet, then extend one leg back at a time until both legs are straight and you are in a plank position, with your shoulders over your hands. Hold for a moment. Reverse the move by bringing each foot toward your hands to return to the squat position, then driving up through your hips to return to a standing position. Repeat quickly for 2 minutes.

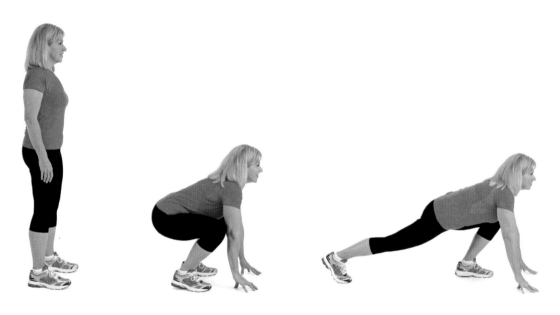

MAKE A DIFFERENCE IN 20 MINUTES
Elevate Your Burn

By now you know that when faced with the choice of stairs or elevator, you should always choose the stairs. But what about choosing the stairs over sitting? Take 20 minutes on your lunch break to climb the stairs in your building and burn up to 180 calories in just 20 minutes. That's a huge calorie burn for only 20 minutes of huffing and puffing.

Tips

- If you have restricted movement in your hips, begin with your legs in a wider stance.

- It's very important to focus on keeping your navel pulled toward your spine in the plank position—do not allow your back to arch.

FEEL THE BURN

To increase your calorie burn, add jumps: Replace the step back and the step in with a jump back and a jump in. If you really want to up the cardiovascular intensity and upper-body workout, you can also add a pushup from the plank position before you return to standing.

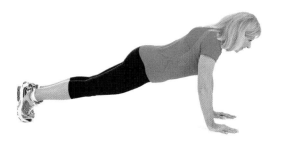

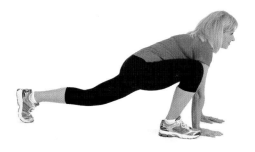

HIGH KNEES

Stand with your feet under your hips and your arms by your sides. Start marching in place and progress to a light jog in place, allowing your arms to swing naturally by your sides. Keeping your abdominals engaged, lean back slightly and begin to lift your knees high in front of you. Continue for 2 minutes.

Tips

- Keep your chest lifted and your neck relaxed.
- Stay light on your feet by thinking of lifting up, rather than pounding into your legs.

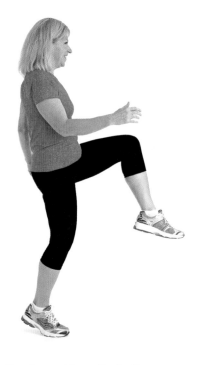

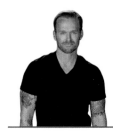 **Biggest Loser Trainer Tip: Bob Harper**

Studies show that having support from your friends and family is crucial to weight-loss success. *Biggest Loser* Club is an online Web site where you have access to friends and experts 24/7. You'll find advice, tips, and all the support you need to make sure your weight-loss journey stays on track.

Log on to **www.biggestloserclub.com**

SKATER

Stand with your feet together and your arms by your sides. Step one leg out to the side in as wide a stance as possible. With your right foot, step diagonally to the left side, leaving your left leg bent at the knee. Allow your body to rotate slightly toward the stepping leg and your arms to move naturally. Gradually pick up the tempo and increase the distance of your steps. Continue for 2 minutes.

Tips

- To allow for greater range of motion, keep your knees bent as you increase your speed.
- Allow your torso to hinge forward slightly as the width of your steps increases. Keep your abdominals pulled in to protect your lower back.
- Maintain proper alignment by keeping the knee of the stepping leg over the ankle.

FEEL THE BURN

To dial up your aerobic workout, increase your speed and change the step to a small jump, landing gently with knees bent. For a really intense burn, keep your back foot off the floor as you leap from side to side. (It's okay to slow down a little so you don't lose your balance!)

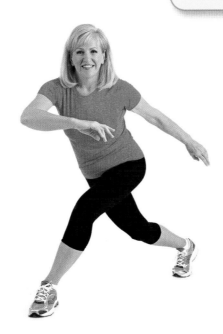

MOUNTAIN CLIMBER

Begin in a plank position with your shoulders over your hands and your legs fully extended behind you. Pull one knee in toward your chest, so that you are on your toes with one leg extended behind you and the other bent underneath you. In one quick motion, switch legs, keeping your upper torso still and your abdominals engaged. Repeat quickly for 2 minutes.

Tips

- Keep the proper shoulder-over-hand alignment so that you can safely use your arm, chest, and back muscles to support your upper body.

- Actively pull your abdominals up and in.

- Keep your core engaged by pushing away from the floor rather than collapsing down.

- Focus on pulling in your knee rather than extending your leg. This will engage your abdominal muscles more fully and protect your feet and ankles.

FEEL THE BURN

The Mountain Climber already provides a vigorous cardio workout when performed properly. But if you want to really get your heart pounding, try going even faster.

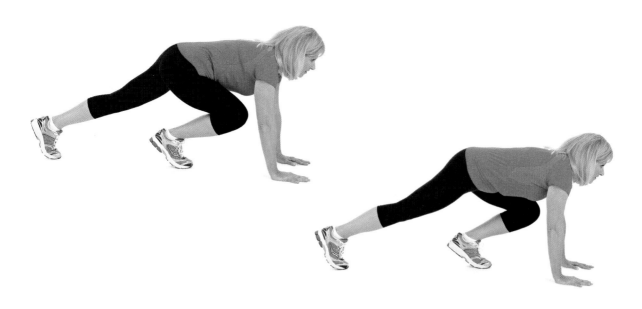

20-Minute Fitness for Advanced Exercisers: Workout 2 (All Strength Training)

The exercises that follow target your lower body and your upper body. You will need a set of dumbbells to complete this circuit. Use a weight that is comfortable for you but still challenging. For some of these exercises, you'll also need an exercise mat or yoga mat, or you can simply use the floor in a carpeted area of your home.

Once you've completed one circuit of these 10 exercises, complete a second circuit, for a total of 20 minutes of strength training.

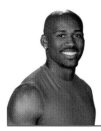

Biggest Loser Trainer Tip: Dolvett Quince

It's so important to stay hydrated when you're working out. I always urge my contestants to drink coconut water in addition to plain water. It rehydrates you quickly. Just make sure not to overindulge—it does contain calories.

SQUAT

Holding a dumbbell in each hand, stand with your feet shoulder-width apart, toes pointing forward, arms by your sides. Keep your chest lifted, spine neutral, and your abdominal muscles engaged. Send your hips back and bend your knees as if you were sitting in a chair, until your thighs are parallel to the floor. Push into your heels to return to the starting position. Do 12 to 15 repetitions.

Tips

- Keep your spine neutral and avoid rounding your back.
- Don't let the dumbbells swing past your shins; aim them straight down toward the floor.

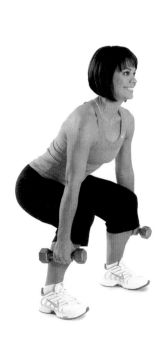
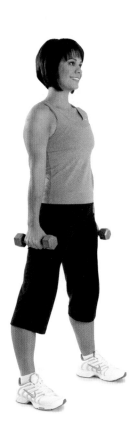

REAR LUNGE

Holding a dumbbell in each hand, stand with your feet together, toes pointing forward, and arms by your sides. Step back with your right leg as far as possible and bend both knees until your left thigh is parallel to the floor. Press into your left foot and bring your right leg forward to return to the starting position. Do 12 to 15 reps, then switch legs and repeat.

Tips

- Keep the shin of the front leg perpendicular to the floor, with your knee directly over your ankle. Don't let your knee move past your toes.

- Maintain a neutral spine, with your shoulders over your hips.

- Keep your arms by your sides to avoid swinging the dumbbells.

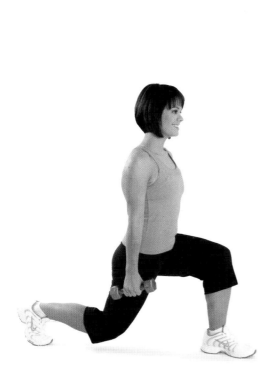
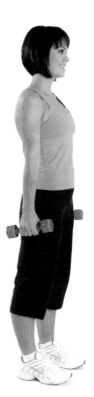

SIDE LUNGE

Holding a dumbbell in each hand, stand with your feet together and your arms by your sides. Step out to the side with your left leg as far as you can (2 to 3 feet) and bend your left knee until your thigh is parallel to the ground. Keep your right leg straight and your spine neutral. Allow your torso to hinge forward slightly as you send your hips back. Press into your left foot and return to the starting position. Do 12 to 15 repetitions, then switch legs and repeat.

Tips

- Hold the dumbbells by your sides as you begin, and as you step out into the lunge, place them at the sides of your bending knee.

- Maintain a neutral spine and a lifted chest throughout this exercise.

FEEL THE BURN

Increase the burn in your second circuit by increasing the weight of your dumbbells slightly. If you started with 5-pound dumbbells, you could bump it up to 6- or 7-pound weights. Just be sure that extra weight doesn't compromise your form. As with all strength training, it's more important to do the exercises correctly than to do them with heavy weights.

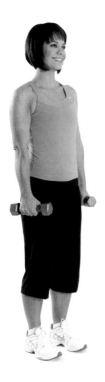

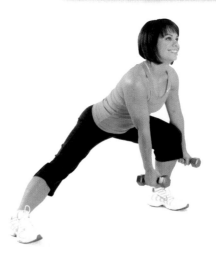

BENT-OVER ROW

Begin in a staggered stance with your left leg forward and your right leg back. Hold a dumbbell in your right hand, with your palm facing in. Bend both knees and hinge slightly forward from the hips, placing your left hand on your left thigh. Keeping your spine neutral and your abdominal muscles engaged, pull the dumbbell up toward your chest, squeezing the muscles in your upper back. Hold for a moment, then lower the dumbbell. Do 12 to 15 repetitions, then switch sides and repeat.

Tips

- Avoid rounding your back.
- Control the movement and don't allow your elbow to lock when you lower the dumbbell.
- Keep your navel pulled in and your abdominals engaged at all times.

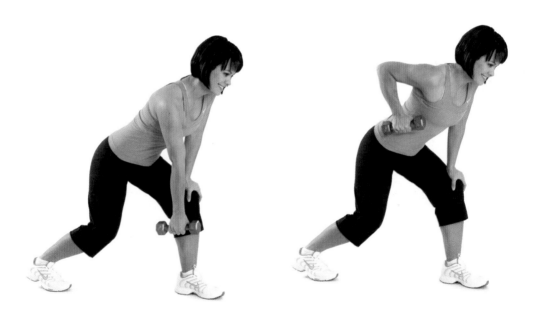

ROMANIAN DEAD LIFT

Holding a dumbbell in each hand, stand with your feet shoulder-width apart, toes pointing forward, and arms by your sides. Keeping your knees slightly bent, bend at the hips, extending your arms toward your toes, until your back is parallel to the floor. Don't allow your back to round. Engage your glutes and abdominal muscles to return to the starting position. Do 12 to 15 repetitions.

Tips

- Maintain a neutral spine and pull your shoulder blades together throughout the exercise.
- Bend only at the hips, not at the spine.
- If your hamstrings are tight and your back begins to round, bend your knees a bit more.

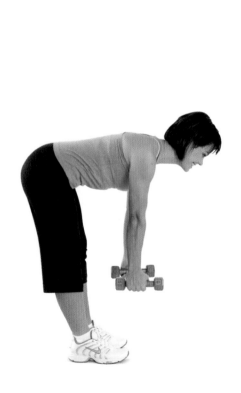 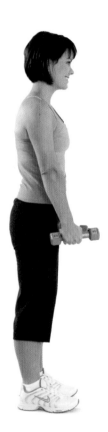

PLIE SQUAT

Holding a dumbbell in each hand, stand with your feet wider than your hips (2 to 3 feet apart), with your legs rotated out from your hips so that your toes point out to the sides (think 2 and 10 o'clock). Place your hands on your hips or in front of your thighs. Bend your knees and lower your hips and torso toward the floor, keeping your back neutral and chest lifted. Make sure that your knees are aligned over your feet and that they do not go past your toes. Press into the floor and return to the starting position. Do 12 to 15 reps.

Tips

- Don't allow your body to shift forward or backward as you bend your knees.
- Imagine lengthening your spine as you squat.
- Rotate from the hips, not the knees or ankles.

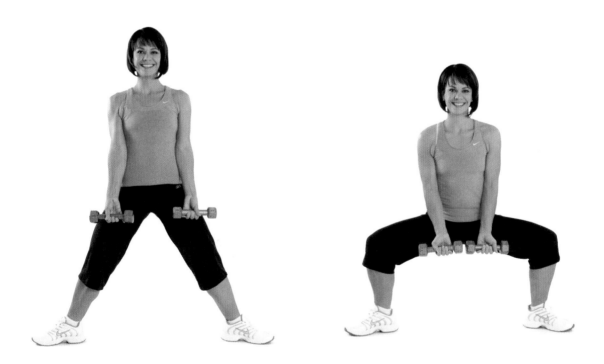

CHEST PRESS

Lie on your back on an exercise mat or a carpeted surface with your knees bent, feet flat on the floor, and toes pointing forward. Hold one dumbbell in each hand directly over your chest, with your arms extended straight up and your palms facing your thighs so that you can see the backs of your hands. Slowly bend your elbows and lower your arms out to your sides, stopping just before your arms touch the floor. Hold for a moment, then press up to the starting position. Do 12 to 15 repetitions.

Tips

- Maintain a neutral spine and don't let your back arch as you bend your elbows.
- Keep the dumbbells over your chest, not your face.

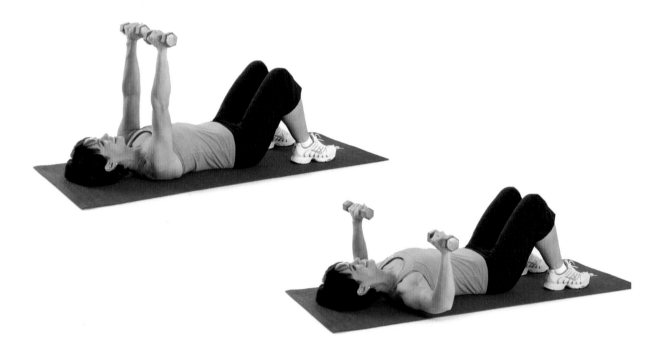

BICEPS CURL

Stand with your feet shoulder-width apart and your toes pointing forward. Hold a dumbbell in each hand, with your arms by your sides and your palms facing in. Slowly bend your elbows and bring the dumbbells up toward your shoulders as you rotate your wrists so that your palms face you. Squeeze your biceps and hold for a moment. Return to the starting position. Do 12 to 15 repetitions.

Tips

- Keep your elbows slightly in front of your body.
- Don't swing the dumbbells.
- Center your weight over your toes and don't allow your back to arch.

FEEL THE BURN

Challenge your balance by standing on one leg during this exercise. You'll engage your core muscles and your lower body as well as your upper body.

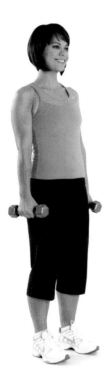
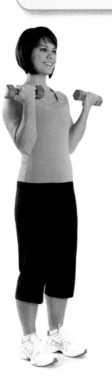

TRICEPS EXTENSION

Begin in a staggered stance with your left leg forward and your right leg back. Hold a dumbbell in your right hand, with your palm facing in. Bend both knees and hinge slightly forward from the hips, placing your left hand on your left thigh. Keeping your spine neutral and your abdominal muscles engaged, pull the dumbbell up toward your chest, squeezing the muscles in your upper back. Keeping your upper arm in this position, slowly extend your elbow as you press the dumbbell back in an arc until your arm is parallel to the floor. Squeeze the back of your upper arm, then slowly bend at the elbow. Do 12 to 15 repetitions, then switch sides and repeat.

Tips

- Keep your abdominal muscles engaged and don't allow your back to arch or round.

- Keep your neck long and roll your shoulders down and back, away from your ears.

- Think of extending your arm out and back, rather than just up.

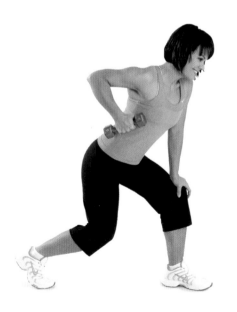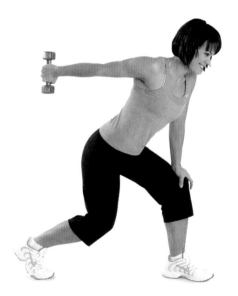

OVERHEAD PRESS

Stand with your feet shoulder-width apart and toes pointing forward. Hold a dumbbell in each hand, near your shoulders, with your elbows bent and palms facing forward. Press the dumbbells upward until your arms are extended overhead. Hold for a moment, then lower the weights to the starting position. Do 12 to 15 repetitions.

Tips

- Maintain a neutral spine and avoid arching your back.

- Try not to lean forward or backward.

- If there's too much tension in your neck, press your arms up in a slightly forward diagonal, rather than straight overhead.

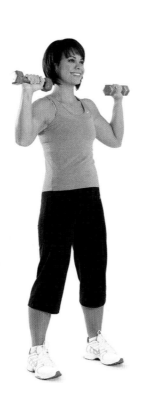
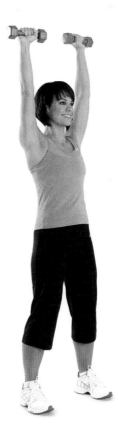

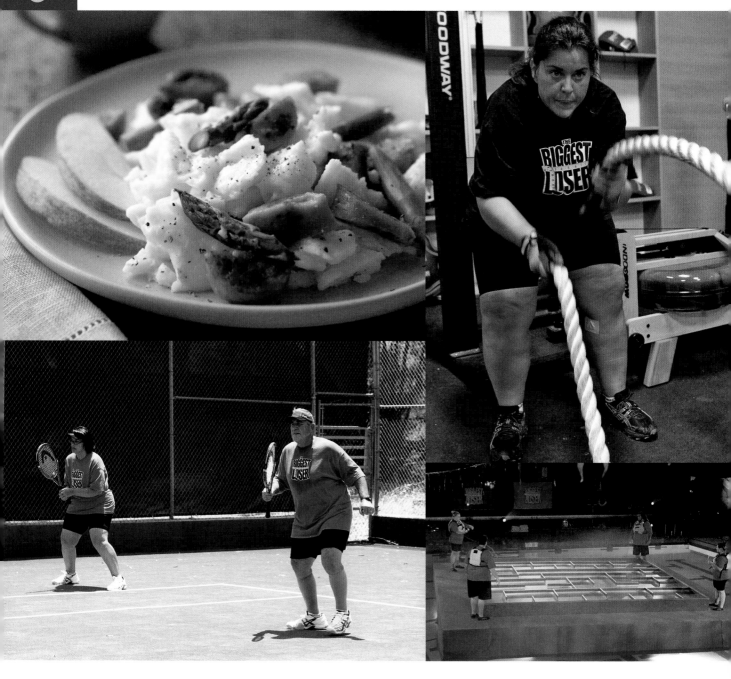

Breakfast on the Double

You've heard it a million times: Breakfast is the most important meal of the day. We all know we're supposed to eat breakfast, but a lot of us still aren't doing it. Most mornings, we barely have time to grab coffee on our way out the door. And besides, *why* is it so important, anyway? Doesn't skipping a meal save calories?

It turns out there's some powerful evidence in favor of fueling up in the a.m. In fact, eating within an hour of waking up helps to jump-start your metabolism, which will help you to burn more calories throughout the day. If you don't snack after dinner and get at least 8 hours of sleep at night, your body's likely been fasting for about 15 hours, which means it's not producing the enzymes needed to metabolize fat—that is, until you feed it again.

Eating early in the day—ideally a meal that includes a combination of fiber, whole grains, and protein—also keeps your blood sugar level stable, preventing you from experiencing that shaky, hungry feeling that can strike mid-morning and send you headfirst into a pile of jelly doughnuts.

"Managing your weight isn't only about cutting calories. It's also about getting more of the good stuff you need, like whole grains," advises *Biggest Loser* trainer Bob Harper. Bob regularly encourages the contestants to eat a healthy breakfast. "Studies show that people who eat more whole grain tend to have healthier body weights," he adds.

Some studies have also shown that regular breakfast eaters are more likely to exercise regularly and to eat less overall calories in a day. Additionally, eating breakfast is a daily habit of people who have lost

30 or more pounds and successfully kept it off long term, according to The National Weight Control Registry.

If you work out in the morning, it's a good idea to split your breakfast into two mini-meals. Try to eat a small snack that's easy on your stomach—such as a banana with a little peanut butter or a half-serving of oatmeal with berries—before you hit the gym, to give you the energy you need for your workout. After your workout, it's important to eat some protein to help your muscles recover. Good choices include a low-calorie protein drink or scrambled egg whites with a slice of Canadian bacon.

Season 9's Cheryl George says the one food she learned to love on the Ranch was protein-rich Greek yogurt. "I like to mix it with cereal and berries for a quick breakfast or a snack," she says.

So what are you waiting for? From Margherita Breakfast Pizza (page 78) to Chocolate Pomegranate Protein Oatmeal (page 81), Chef Devin gives you several quick, easy, and delicious reasons to start off your day on the right foot.

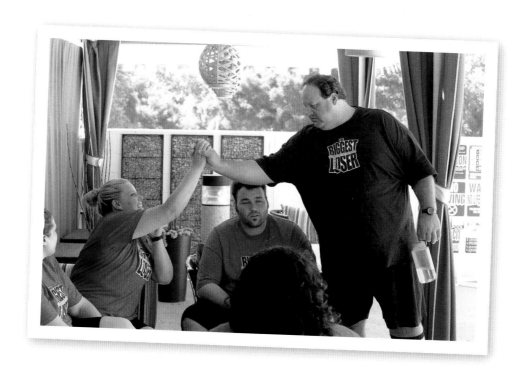

FLORENTINE BREAKFAST QUESADILLA

For years, The Biggest Loser *trainers and nutritionists have emphasized the importance of starting your day with a healthy breakfast. If you can incorporate veggies into your morning meal, all the better. The more veggies you eat, and the earlier in the day you eat them, the less likely you'll be to face cravings as the day progresses.*

1 (10") all-natural sprouted grain tortilla or other (8") all-natural, low-fat whole grain tortilla (I used French Meadow Bakery Organic Sprouted Grain Tortillas)

1 ounce (about ⅓ cup) finely shredded all-natural, low-fat Cheddar cheese (I used Cabot's 75% Reduced Fat Sharp Cheddar Cheese)

Olive oil spray (propellant free)

½ cup 100% liquid egg whites

½ cup fresh spinach leaves

Place a nonstick frying pan, large enough for the tortilla to lie flat, over medium-low heat. Put the tortilla in the pan. Sprinkle the cheese evenly over the tortilla. Let the cheese melt for 2 to 4 minutes.

Meanwhile, place a small nonstick pan over medium-high heat. Lightly mist it with the olive oil spray and add the egg substitute. As the eggs begin to set, use a wooden spoon to scrape from one side of the pan to the other, to scramble them. Continue scrambling until no runny egg remains.

Add the spinach leaves and cook, stirring constantly, for 30 seconds, or until the spinach is just wilted. Spoon the egg mixture over the cheese on half of the tortilla. Fold the tortilla in half. Transfer the quesadilla to a cutting board and cut it into 4 wedges. Serve immediately.

Makes 1 serving

Per serving: 285 calories, 32 g protein, 29 g carbohydrates (2 g sugar), 3 g fat, 2 g saturated fat, 10 mg cholesterol, 6 g fiber, 582 mg sodium

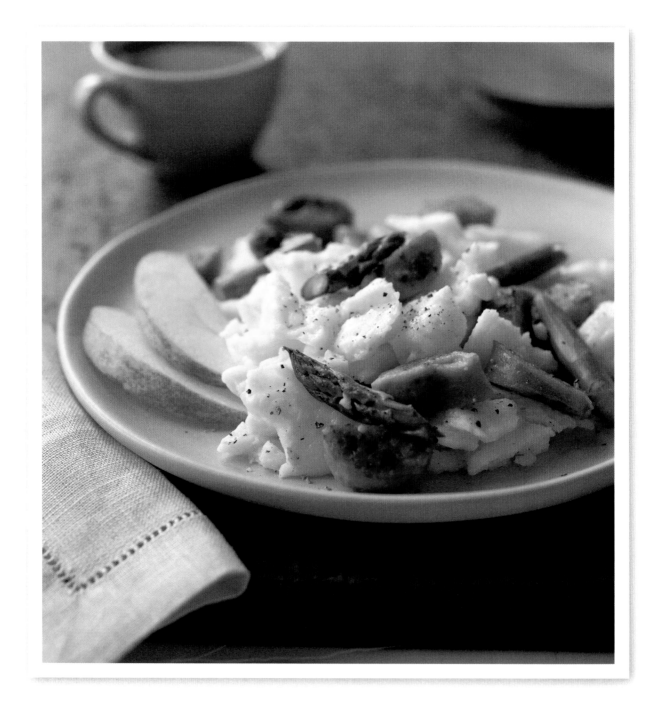

ASPARAGUS AND CHICKEN APPLE SAUSAGE SCRAMBLE

Dishes like this scramble can really start your day off on the right foot. You're nourishing your body with a significant serving of food for very few calories, and it's satisfying to be able to enjoy breakfast "classics" like eggs and sausage. Just be sure to read the label when you shop for sausage. You want to find one that's nitrate free and as low in fat and salt as possible.

Olive oil spray (propellant free)

4 large egg whites

2 ounces all-natural nitrate-free chicken and apple sausage, cut into bite-size cubes

4 large asparagus spears, trimmed and cut into 1" pieces

Sea salt, to taste

Fresh ground black pepper, to taste

Coat a medium microwave-safe bowl with the olive oil spray. Add the egg whites.

Preheat a small nonstick skillet over medium heat. Lightly mist it with the spray. When hot, add the sausage and asparagus and cook, stirring often, for 4 to 7 minutes, or until the asparagus is crisp-tender and the sausage is lightly browned.

Meanwhile, microwave the egg whites for 30 seconds on low heat. Continue microwaving them in 30-second intervals until they are just a bit runny on top. Stir them with a fork, breaking them apart into large pieces. By the time you "scramble" and stir them, the residual heat should have cooked away the runniness. If they are still runny, cook them in 10-second intervals until just done.

Add the cooked sausage and asparagus mixture to the egg whites and mix well with a fork. Season with salt and pepper and serve immediately.

Makes 1 serving

Per serving: 185 calories, 25 g protein, 10 g carbohydrates (7 g sugar), 6 g fat, 2 g saturated fat, 42 mg cholesterol, 2 g fiber, 507 mg sodium

SAUSAGE FETA PEPPER BAKE

I love breakfast dishes like this one. They are extremely low in calories for their serving size, and they allow me (and, more important, you!) to couple them with a low-fat muffin, a small smoothie, or a bowl of fruit and still stay under 350 calories for the whole meal.

Olive oil spray (propellant free)

4 ounces lean nitrate-free spinach and feta chicken and/or turkey sausage, sliced lengthwise and then chopped into ½" pieces (no more than 7 grams of fat per 3-ounce link)

2 cups frozen pepper and onion blend

2 cups all-natural egg substitute

Sea salt, to taste

Fresh ground black pepper, to taste

Preheat the oven to 400°F.

Place a medium oven-safe nonstick skillet over high heat. Lightly mist the pan with the olive oil spray and add the sausage and pepper blend. Cook for 4 to 6 minutes, or until all of the moisture is cooked away and the onions, peppers, and sausage are lightly browned.

Turn the heat off and pour the egg substitute into the pan. Transfer the pan to the oven and bake for 12 to 14 minutes, or until the eggs are completely set. Season with the salt and pepper. Being careful not to scratch your pan, cut into four equal wedges and serve immediately.

Makes 4 servings

Per serving: 113 calories, 17 g protein, 5 g carbohydrates (4 g sugar), 2 g fat, <1 g saturated fat, 20 mg cholesterol, trace fiber, 412 mg sodium

Becky Comet SEASON 12

Keep a food journal. It's difficult to know where to start nutritionally if you don't know what you're putting in your body on a daily basis. Statistics show that people who keep a food journal have more lasting success in weight loss.

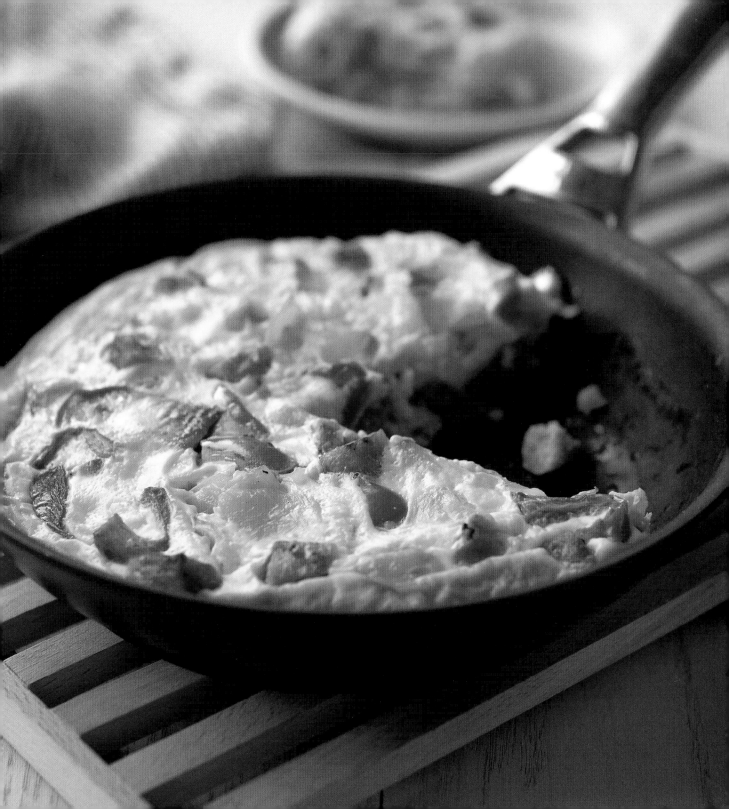

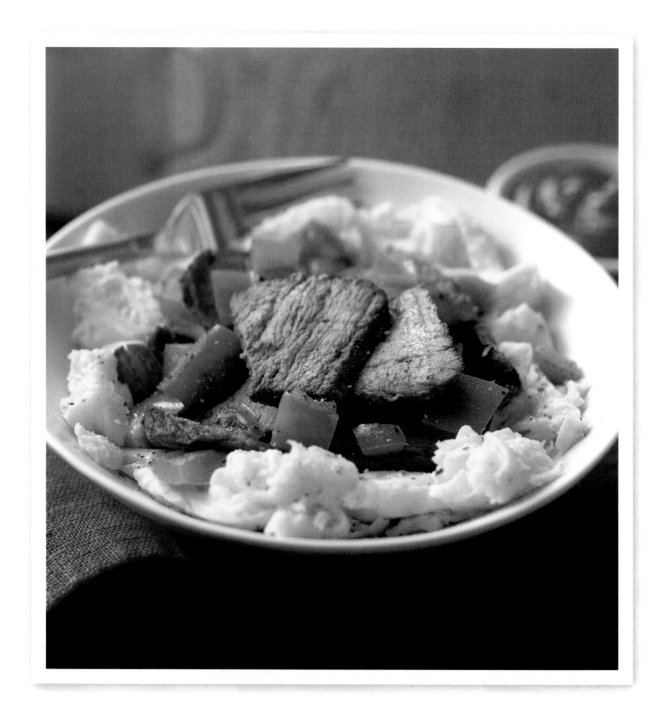

STEAK AND EGG BREAKFAST BOWL

Steak and Eggs is a breakfast favorite of many Biggest Loser *contestants prior to their arrival at the Ranch. After hearing a number of them say, "I'd kill to have steak and eggs for breakfast," I came up with this yummy, simple dish to satisfy their cravings without blowing their calorie budgets.*

To save even more time, you can microwave the eggs (you'd be surprised how light and fluffy the microwave makes them). For a spicier twist on this dish, you can always top it with a fresh salsa or salsa verde. Or, if you like really spicy foods, add a dash of hot sauce.

Olive oil spray (propellant free)

3 ounces trimmed top round steak or London broil, cut into bite-size strips

½ large green bell pepper, coarsely chopped (about ⅓ cup)

½ cup all-natural egg substitute

All-natural ketchup, preferably agave or honey sweetened and low in salt, to taste (optional)

Place a medium nonstick skillet over high heat. When the skillet is hot, lightly mist it with the olive oil spray. Add the steak and pepper in a single layer. Cook, stirring occasionally, for 2 to 3 minutes, or until the pepper is crisp-tender and the steak is browned on the outside and cooked to desired doneness.

Meanwhile, place a small nonstick skillet over medium heat. Mist the skillet lightly with the spray and add the egg substitute. When the eggs are slightly set, scrape the bottom of the skillet with a wooden spoon to scramble them. Repeat until the eggs are cooked.

Spoon the egg mixture into a bowl. Top it with the steak and pepper mixture. Serve immediately with the ketchup, if desired.

Makes 1 serving

Per serving: **161 calories, 31 g protein, 6 g carbohydrates (4 g sugar), 3 g fat, 1 g saturated fat, 38 mg cholesterol, 1 g fiber, 294 mg sodium**

OPEN-FACE GOURMET ITALIAN BREAKFAST SANDWICH

We all know that going to the drive-thru is not an option for breakfast, but that doesn't mean you can't enjoy a delicious breakfast sandwich. If you choose wisely, it can be an extremely sensible breakfast choice. In previous books, I've written recipes for the traditional egg, sausage, and cheese breakfast sandwich. To change things up, I'm taking you on a bit more of a gourmet ride with another of my favorite breakfast sandwiches that starts out your day with a healthy dose of greens.

Olive oil spray (propellant free)

2 large egg whites

½ all-natural, low-fat whole grain English muffin (I used Rudi's Organic Bakery Whole Grain Wheat English Muffins)

1 slice (about ⅔ ounce) reduced-fat provolone cheese

1 slice (about ½ ounce) nitrite-free turkey salami (I used Applegate Uncured Turkey Salami)

¼ cup arugula

Lightly mist a 3½"- or 4"-diameter microwave-safe bowl or ramekin with the olive oil spray. Add the egg whites. Microwave them for 30 seconds, then continue microwaving them in 15-second intervals until they are just set (do not stir them).

Meanwhile, toast the English muffin in a toaster or under the broiler.

Assemble the sandwich by placing the English muffin, cut side up, on a plate. Top it, in order, with the cheese, eggs, salami, and arugula. Serve immediately.

Makes 1 sandwich

Per sandwich: 166 calories, 17 g protein, 13 g carbohydrates (2 g sugar), 5 g fat, 2 g saturated fat, 20 mg cholesterol, 2 g fiber, 487 mg sodium

Johnny Forger SEASON 12

Your past? Forget about it! It's over. This is a *new* lifestyle. Remember that every day. This is a great way to live—to be healthy and happy. Focus on those thoughts and be patient. It's all going to happen.

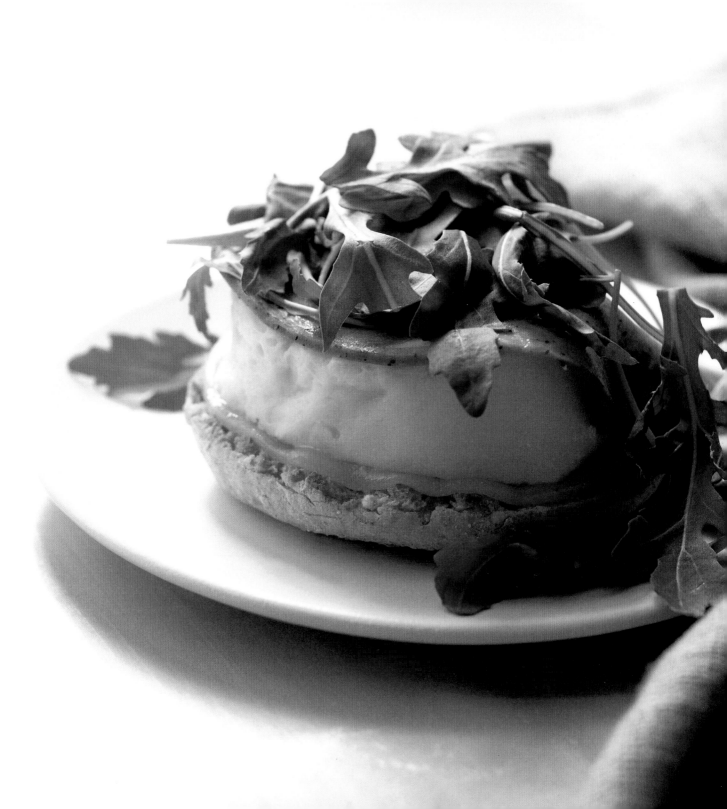

MARGHERITA BREAKFAST PIZZA

Many, many years ago, I figured out that you can crisp a flour tortilla to make an excellent thin pizza crust. In the years following my TV appearances demonstrating this, I noticed a ton of other chefs doing this as well. Yet 10-plus years ago, everyone was making English muffin pizzas—those were the common fallback. Here I've "returned to the old days" with a breakfast version of one of the most traditional pizzas ever.

1 all-natural, low-fat whole grain English Muffin (I used Rudi's Organic Bakery Whole Grain Wheat English Muffins), split in half

1 ounce (¼ cup) finely shredded almond mozzarella cheese (I used Lisanatti)*

4 medium basil leaves

2 grape tomatoes, quartered, or more to taste

Olive oil spray (propellant free)

Preheat the oven to 450°F.

Place the muffin halves, cut side up, on a small baking sheet. Sprinkle the cheese evenly over both muffin halves. Top the cheese with 2 basil leaves per muffin half, and place the tomatoes on top of the basil. Lightly mist each with the olive oil spray.

Bake for 5 to 7 minutes, until the cheese is melted and the muffin is lightly toasted. Serve immediately.

Makes 1 serving

Per serving: 189 calories, 12 g protein, 28 g carbohydrates (3 g sugar), 3 g fat, trace saturated fat, 0 mg cholesterol, 4 g fiber, 422 mg sodium

When shredding lower-fat cheeses, it's always better to shred them finely. Not only does it take less cheese to cover more surface area, it melts better. That said, Lisanatti just introduced preshredded cheese. If you can find it preshredded, go for it—and don't worry that it's not superfine. The finished dish will still be delish!

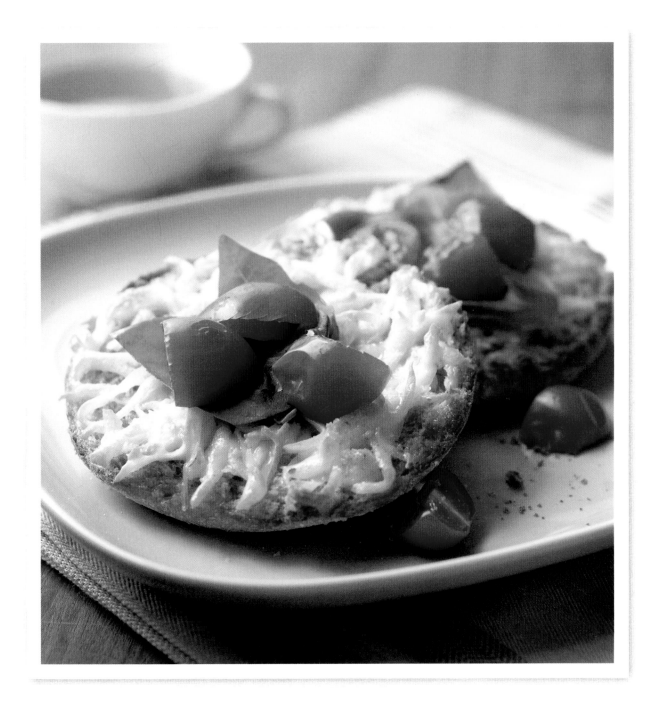

BUFF BLUEBERRY QUINOA

Quinoa, pronounced "keen-wah," is an ancient grain that has become more and more popular in recent years because of its great nutritional value. Though it's often used in savory dishes, it also makes a great base for breakfast dishes. If you haven't tried it yet, now's the time!

1 cup frozen blueberries, thawed

1 teaspoon honey, or more to taste

¾ cup cooked quinoa, reheated if necessary (see Basic Quinoa on page xxiii for cooking instructions)

½ tablespoon chopped dry roasted almonds

Place the blueberries in a medium glass or plastic mixing bowl. Use a potato masher or a pastry blender to thoroughly mash the blueberries and release most of their juice.

Add the honey and quinoa and stir until combined.

Transfer to a serving bowl and top with the almonds. Serve immediately.

Makes 1 serving (scant cup)

Per serving: 277 calories, 8 g protein, 53 g carbohydrates (18 g sugar), 5 g fat, trace saturated fat, 0 mg cholesterol, 8 g fiber, 10 mg sodium

Bonnie Griffin SEASON 12

One morning I was in a rush to work out, so I grabbed a piece of whole wheat bread and toasted it. I topped it with two slices of cooked turkey bacon and sprinkled on a little low-fat Cheddar cheese. It turned out to be a quick, tasty breakfast!

CHOCOLATE POMEGRANATE PROTEIN OATMEAL

If you aren't familiar with pomegranate powder or cacao powder, they are raw superfood powders. They add powerful nutrients and antioxidants to dishes without adding a lot of calories. If you can't find them in stores, you can order them online from Navitas Naturals. This company's powders are certified organic, kosher, vegan, and raw. True, they're a little expensive, but if you plan to add them to oatmeal, smoothies, and even baked goods, you'll likely find them to be a great investment.

½ cup old-fashioned oats

½ scoop (8.5 grams) Biggest Loser All Natural Chocolate Deluxe Protein Supplement (or 25 calories' worth of other chocolate protein powder)

1½ teaspoons pomegranate powder (I used Navitas Naturals Pomegranate Powder)

1 teaspoon cacao or cocoa powder

1 teaspoon light agave nectar, or to taste

In a small saucepan, bring 1 cup water to a rolling boil over high heat. Add the oats and reduce the heat to medium. Cook for 5 to 7 minutes, or until most of the liquid is evaporated. Remove the pan from the heat and cover for 2 to 3 minutes.

Stir in the protein powder, pomegranate powder, cacao, and agave until well combined. Serve immediately.

Makes 1 serving

Per serving: **222 calories, 10 g protein, 41 g carbohydrates (8 g sugar), 3 g fat, trace saturated fat, 10 mg cholesterol, 8 g fiber, 37 mg sodium**

MAKE A DIFFERENCE IN 20 MINUTES
Weight Loss's Best Friend

On a cold or rainy morning, no one feels like taking the family dog for a walk. But the next time your kids and spouse race to say "Not it!" you'll know that just 20 minutes of moderate walking with Fido can buy you 91 calories' worth of breakfast. Not a bad deal for you or your pooch.

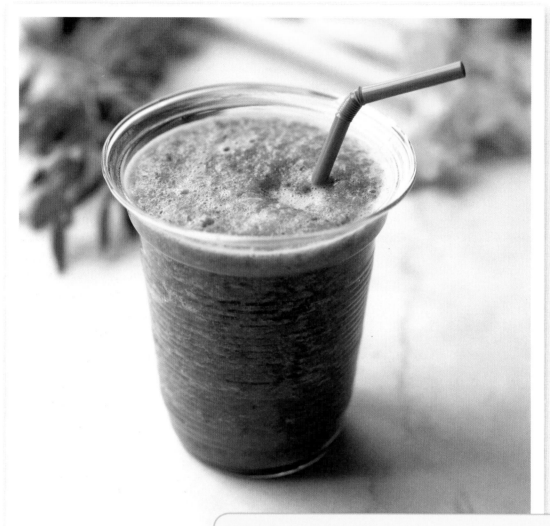

GREENS ON-THE-GO JUICE

"Green" drinks have become quite a trend in recent years. And they can be a great way to get veggies in your diet in a simple, convenient way. This recipe makes a big batch of green juice that you can drink over a few days. I suggest you make it in your blender and don't strain it, to get the maximum benefit. If, however, the pulp bothers you, you can use a rubber spatula to push it through a strainer or you can prepare it in a juicer. Note that straining results in a juice with less fiber, and a juicer removes most, if not all, of the fiber, according to Biggest Loser *medical expert Dr. Dansinger.*

---

1 small cucumber, cut into large cubes

3 cups 100% pink grapefruit juice, not from concentrate

1 bag (5 ounces) fresh spinach leaves

8 stalks celery, trimmed and broken into 4 pieces

4 cups parsley leaves (it's okay if a bit of stem remains)

To the jar of a blender, add the cucumber along with ½ cup of the grapefruit juice. Blend on high speed until smooth. Continuing adding enough spinach, celery, and parsley so that the blender is no more than three-fourths full. Blend on high speed until smooth, stopping the blender intermittently to scrape the sides and press the ingredients into the center if necessary. Continue adding and blending until no veggies remain. (Add some of the remaining grapefruit juice at this stage, *only if necessary* to help the blending process.)

Strain the juice, if desired. Stir in the remaining grapefruit juice.

Divide the juice among 4 glasses (no smaller than 12 ounces) or resealable drinking cups. Serve immediately or refrigerate for up to 2 days.

Makes 4 servings

Per serving: **154 calories, 4 g protein, 36 g carbohydrates (24 g sugar), <1 g fat, trace saturated fat, 0 mg cholesterol, 7 g fiber, 226 mg sodium**

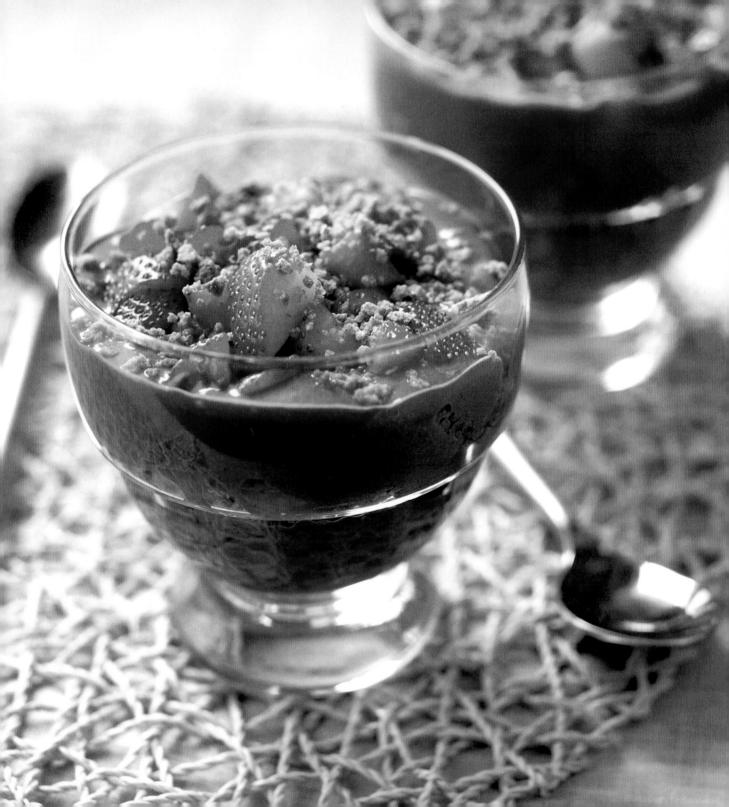

BITTERSWEET CHOCOLATE STRAWBERRY PARFAIT

Anyone who has talked to me for more than 5 minutes knows that I'm the biggest chocoholic ever! I was inspired to create this dish when a number of yogurt companies came out with chocolate-flavored yogurts that looked tempting but contained a lot of sugar, fat, or chemicals. So I took matters into my own kitchen and simply added cocoa powder to vanilla yogurt. If you love dense, bittersweet chocolate as much as I do, you'll love this parfait. If you're not such a chocoholic, you might want to add the cocoa powder a tablespoon at a time.

Each tablespoon of cocoa powder contains only 10 calories but packs 2 grams of fiber. So, in this case, the more chocolate the merrier!

---

3 tablespoons unsweetened cocoa powder

6 ounces fat-free, preferably fruit juice–sweetened vanilla yogurt

1 cup coarsely chopped strawberries, preferably fresh

2 tablespoons whole grain, crunchy, high-fiber, low-sugar cereal (I used Kashi 7 Whole Grain Nuggets)

In a small mixing bowl, stir the cocoa powder into the yogurt until well combined. Spoon half of the mixture into a 16-ounce parfait glass or to-go cup. Top with half of the strawberries, then 1 tablespoon of the cereal. Repeat the layering with the remaining ingredients. Serve immediately or cover and refrigerate for up to 1 day until ready to enjoy.

Makes 1 serving

Per serving: 256 calories, 15 g protein, 54 g carbohydrates (25 g sugar), 2 g fat, trace saturated fat, 0 mg cholesterol, 11 g fiber, 157 mg sodium

>>> *TAKE IT TO GO!* >>>

Layer this yummy parfait in a resealable plastic container up to a day in advance. Just be sure to keep it refrigerated until you're ready to enjoy it. You can even pop it into your kid's lunch box with an ice pack for a healthy snack or lunchtime treat!

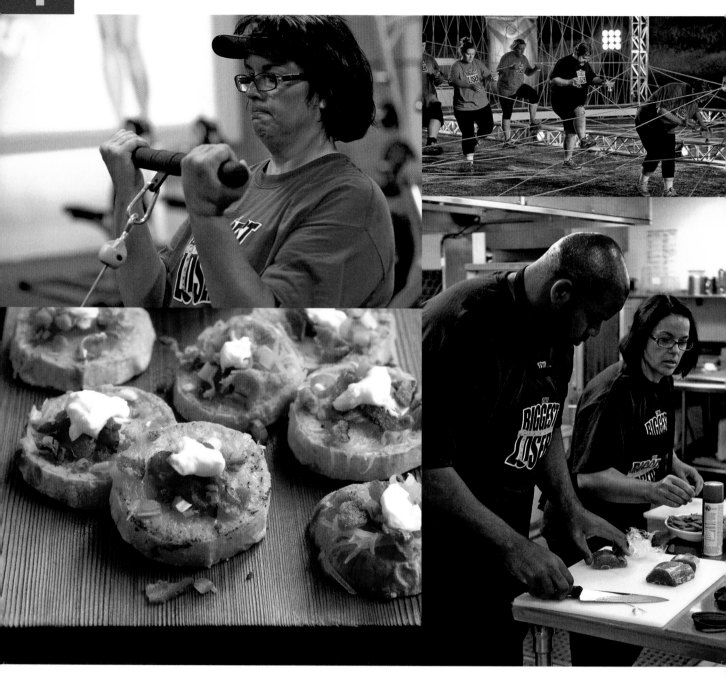

Apps and Snacks, Pronto

Snacks and starters have gotten a bad rap in the world of weight loss. But the truth is, healthy nibbles can go a long way toward helping you reach your weight-loss goals.

Let's look at appetizers. At first glance, they seem like just another course of calories. And at many restaurants, they are. The appetizer menus of many popular chain restaurants are laden with calorie bombs like chicken tenders, egg rolls, and the ever-popular potato skins. These (mostly deep-fried) "starters" can begin your dinner with an entire meal's worth of calories (or more!).

But in the time it takes you to wait for your appetizer order at a restaurant, you can whip up a batch of Pork Notsticker Lettuce Wraps (page 91), Sweet Potato No-Skins (page 94), or Sooo Not Chicken Nuggets (page 107). Each of these apps will help you (and your tastebuds) feel satisfied by the time you get

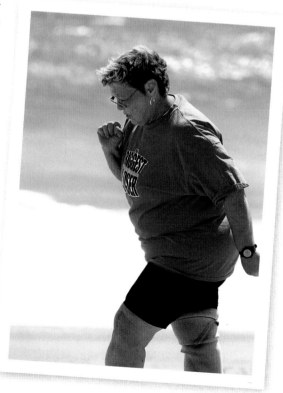

to the end of your meal. Remember, weight loss is not about deprivation—it's about healthy choices.

Snacking is a major weapon in your weight-loss arsenal. Healthy, well-planned snacks keep your blood sugar stable, prevent you from grazing on high-calorie junk food, and give you the energy you need to get in a killer workout.

Season 6's Ed Brantley advises keeping portable snacks on hand at all times. "I keep fresh, cut-up fruit in resealable bags for ready-to-go snacks, along with hard-boiled eggs and containers of yogurt. These are great, powerful foods that can get you through the morning."

On *The Biggest Loser* plan, you should aim to eat your snacks mid-morning and mid-afternoon—two times when hunger always seems to strike. Preplanning your snacks and keeping them handy in the fridge, or brown-bagging them to work, will help you stay on track.

Season 11's Kaylee Kinikini admits that late-night snacking used to be a problem for her. Now, she says, "I stay away from the kitchen late at night. My advice is to just go to bed or distract yourself, read a book or something, because it's not worth it. You'll get into trouble!"

Of course, a simple piece of fruit or some veggies with a little protein (apple slices and peanut butter, carrot sticks and hummus) make an easy snack anytime. But if you're getting a little bored with your tried-and-true healthy snacks, Chef Devin's quick and easy recipes are sure to satisfy.

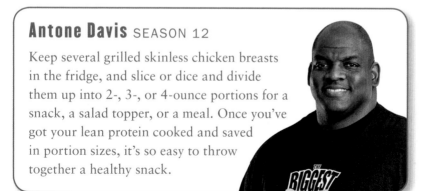

Antone Davis SEASON 12

Keep several grilled skinless chicken breasts in the fridge, and slice or dice and divide them up into 2-, 3-, or 4-ounce portions for a snack, a salad topper, or a meal. Once you've got your lean protein cooked and saved in portion sizes, it's so easy to throw together a healthy snack.

CRAB-STUFFED BELL PEPPERS

Bob, Dolvett, and Anna are always making sure that contestants get plenty of protein and vegetables in their diets and stay away from empty carbs. This recipe is an excellent example of a power snack. The crab provides protein as well as much-needed omega 3 fatty acids. This filling comes together in minutes. Then simply spread it on the bell pepper halves and crunch away! Be sure to use real crab, not the imitation stuff.

3   tablespoons very finely chopped sweet onion

3   tablespoons very finely chopped celery

2   tablespoons all-natural light sandwich spread (I used Spectrum Naturals Light Canola Mayo)

2   teaspoons all-natural prepared horseradish

½   teaspoon salt-free Cajun or creole seasoning (I used The Spice Hunter Salt Free Cajun Creole Seasoning Blend)

8   ounces jumbo lump crabmeat, drained if necessary

2   small green bell peppers, cut in half and seeded

In a medium glass or plastic mixing bowl, mix the onion, celery, sandwich spread, horseradish, and seasoning. Gently stir in the crab until just combined, being careful not to break it too much.

Place 2 pepper halves on each of 2 serving plates. Spoon a quarter of the crab into each half. Serve immediately.

Makes 2 servings

Per serving: 155 calories, 24 g protein, 6 g carbohydrates (3 g sugar), 4 g fat, 1 g saturated fat, 147 mg cholesterol, 2 g fiber, 470 mg sodium

Debbie Lounds SEASON 12

I love Greek yogurt with fresh berries and a touch of Truvía. That snack is less than 200 calories and very filling. I used to not like Greek yogurt, but now I love it!

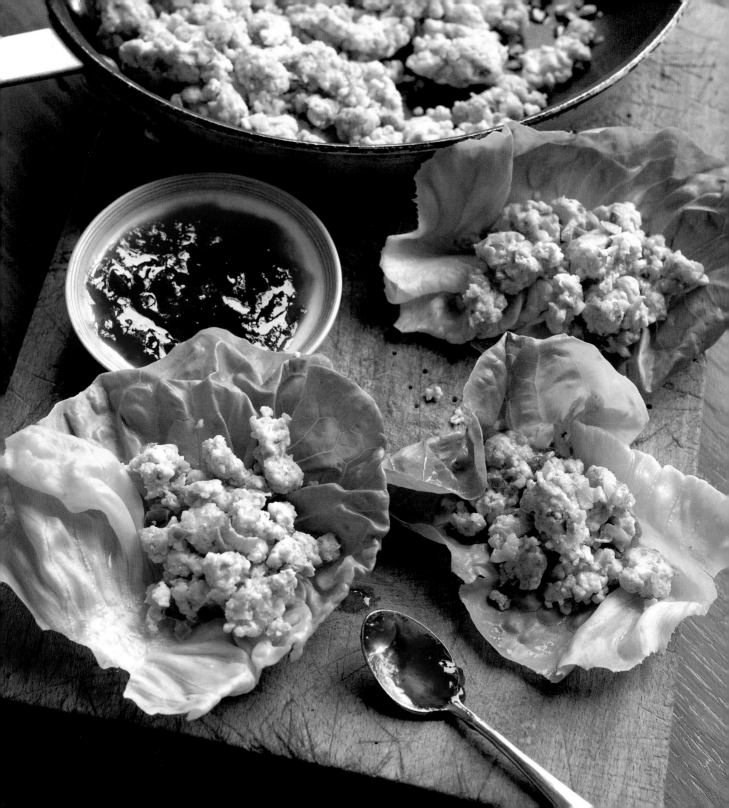

PORK NOTSTICKER LETTUCE WRAPS

In the first Biggest Loser Cookbook, *I worked with former* Biggest Loser *contestants Kimmi Dove and Bruce Lebowsky on their rendition of Kimmi and Bruce's Chicken Lettuce Wraps. Here's another version of this extremely popular dish found in many Asian restaurants. Though I used pork this time, the dish is still exceptionally lean. I even created a dipping sauce with 100 percent natural ingredients!*

4 tablespoons all-natural 100% fruit plum spread (St. Dalfour Fancy Plum 100% Fruit)

1 pound extra-lean ground pork

8 whole small scallions (or 4 medium ones), trimmed and very finely chopped

¼ cup all-natural egg substitute

¼ cup whole wheat panko-style bread crumbs

2 medium cloves garlic, very finely chopped (about 2 teaspoons)

2 teaspoons hot sesame oil

⅛ teaspoon salt

⅛ teaspoon fresh ground black pepper

Olive oil spray (propellant free)

2 tablespoons all-natural, reduced-sodium soy sauce

18 Boston lettuce leaves

Place the plum spread in a small microwave-safe bowl.

In a medium glass or plastic mixing bowl, mix the pork, scallions, egg substitute, bread crumbs, garlic, oil, salt, and pepper until well combined.

Place a large nonstick skillet over medium-high heat. When hot, lightly mist it with the olive oil spray and add the pork mixture to the pan. With a wooden spoon, cook the meat, breaking it into large chunks as you do, for 5 to 8 minutes, or until no longer pink inside.

Meanwhile, microwave the plum spread on medium power for 20 seconds, or until melted. Stir in the soy sauce until well combined.

Put 3 tablespoons of the pork in the center of each lettuce leaf. Top each evenly with 1 teaspoon of the plum sauce.

Makes 6 (3-leaf) servings

Per serving: **190 calories, 19 g protein, 14 g carbohydrates (9 g sugar), 4 g fat, 1 g saturated fat, 50 mg cholesterol, 1 g fiber, 272 mg sodium**

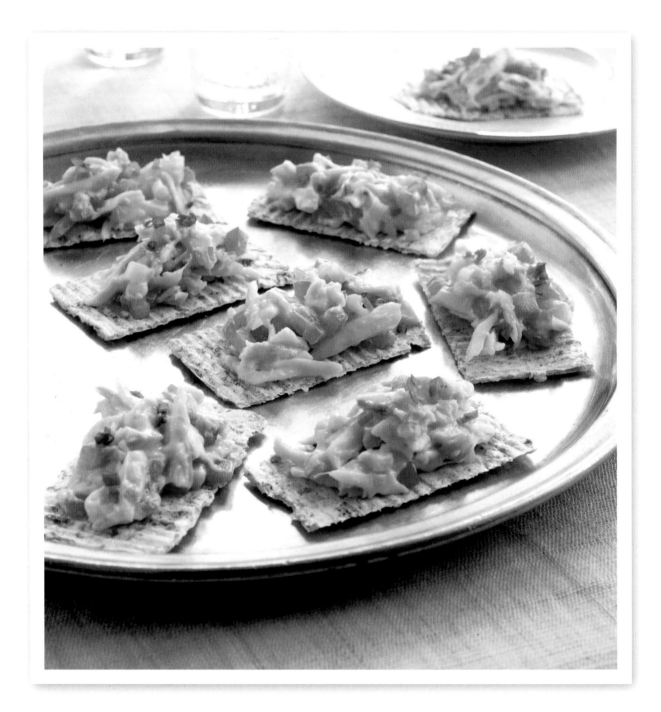

ASIAN CRAB SALAD–TOPPED BROWN RICE CRISPS

I love the elegance of this appetizer when served on round brown rice crackers. You can serve it at fancy events (trust me, I know because I have!), and people will never suspect that they're eating a Biggest Loser*–approved recipe. In fact, they're more likely to think it's really rich, as most crab salads are. This one is just as decadent but way lower in calories!*

The super-crisp brown rice crackers are an excellent choice because they almost seem like they're fried. If you can't find the tamari-seasoned variety, opt for sesame or any other flavor that complements this yummy dish with an Asian flare.

2 whole medium scallions, trimmed and finely chopped (about ⅓ cup)

2 tablespoons all-natural light sandwich spread (I used Spectrum Naturals Light Canola Mayo)

1 teaspoon hot sesame oil

¼ red bell pepper, finely chopped (about ⅓ cup)

8 ounces lump crabmeat, drained if necessary

24 brown rice crackers, preferably tamari-seasoned (I used Edward & Sons Baked Tamari Sesame Brown Rice Snaps)

In a small mixing bowl, stir the scallions, sandwich spread, oil, and pepper until well combined. Gently stir in the crabmeat just until combined. Mound 1 tablespoon of the crab on each cracker. Serve immediately.

Makes 6 (4-cracker) servings

Per serving: 87 calories, 8 g protein, 8 g carbohydrates (trace sugar), 2 g fat, trace saturated fat, 49 mg cholesterol, <1g fiber, 223 mg sodium

>>> TAKE IT TO GO! >>>

To make this a portable snack, pack the crab salad in a resealable plastic container and store it in a cooler bag or the refrigerator. Carry the crackers in a resealable plastic bag. You want to keep the crab salad and the crackers separate until the last minute so the crackers don't become soggy. Scoop the crab with the crackers and enjoy.

SWEET POTATO NO-SKINS

These "No-Skins" incorporate a very strategic use of salt. You season the top of the potato rounds so that when they're flipped, the seasoning will be on the bottom—ensuring that your tongue hits the salt on the potato first! That way, you need less salt overall, and your tastebuds will still be satisfied.

You'll likely fool your children and spouse into thinking these are regular white potatoes if you purchase light-skinned sweet potatoes. Both versions taste delicious, but if you use the darker sweet potatoes, you might need to increase the cooking time a minute or two.

---

16 ounces ½"-thick rounds light-skinned sweet potatoes*

1 teaspoon olive oil

⅛ teaspoon sea salt

⅛ teaspoon garlic powder

⅛ teaspoon cayenne, or to taste

2 ounces finely shredded all-natural, low-fat Cheddar cheese (I used Cabot's 75% Reduced Fat Sharp Cheddar Cheese)

4 teaspoons all-natural bacon bits (I used Wellshire All-Natural Fully Cooked Salt-Cured Bacon Bits)

4 teaspoons finely chopped scallions

2 tablespoons fat-free Greek yogurt (optional)

Preheat the oven to 450°F. Line a baking sheet with nonstick foil.

In a large glass or plastic mixing bowl, toss the potatoes and oil together until the potatoes are well coated.

Place the potato rounds in a single layer on the prepared pan so they do not touch. Sprinkle the salt, garlic powder, and cayenne evenly over the top of the potatoes. Bake them for 10 minutes. Flip them and bake for 7 to 9 minutes longer, or until they are tender inside and starting to brown lightly on the outside.

Push the potato rounds together so that they touch and you can easily top them in a single, even layer. First place the Cheddar, then the bacon bits, and then the scallions over the rounds. Bake for 2 to 3 minutes, or until the cheese is melted. Serve immediately with ½ teaspoon of the yogurt on top of each, if desired.

Makes 4 servings

Per serving: **141 calories, 7 g protein, 21 g carbohydrates (6 g sugar), 3 g fat, 1 g saturated fat, 7 mg cholesterol, 4 g fiber, 283 mg sodium**

You'll need to start with about 1½ pounds of potatoes in order to get 16 ounces of rounds. Try to choose potatoes that are roughly uniform in size. To create the rounds, peel your potatoes and cut both ends off. Then cut them into ½"-thick rounds and measure out 16 ounces.

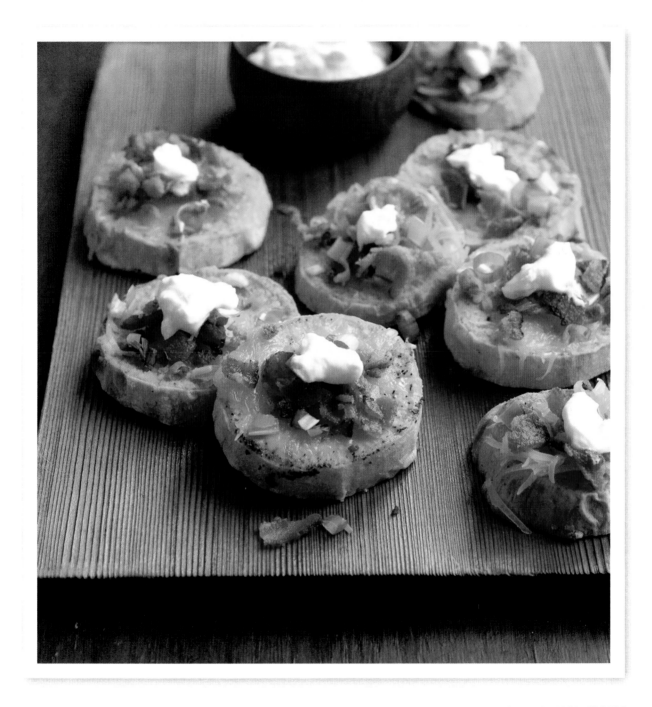

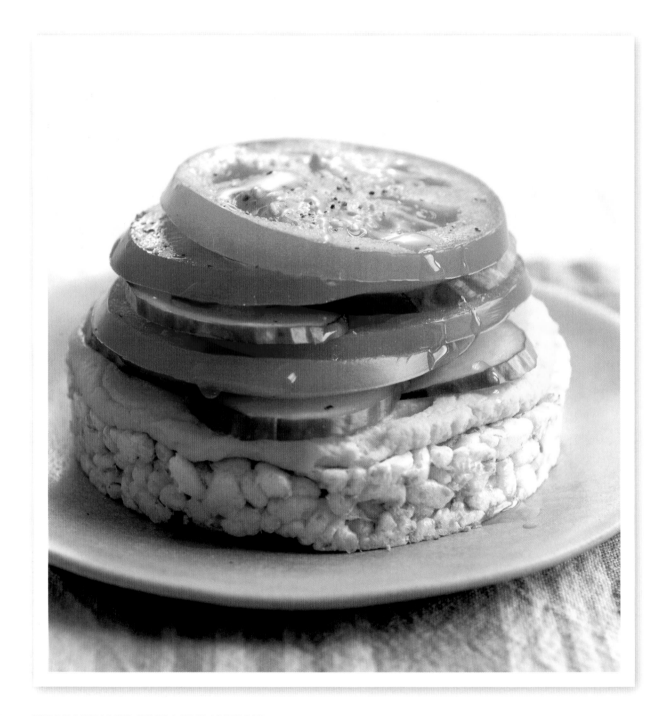

MEDITERRANEAN RICE CAKE STACKER

In recent years, I've become a big fan of seasoned oils. They pack a burst of flavor that can really take a dish from okay to special. I always recommend going to a specialty store where you can sample the olive oils. That way, you can invest in one you know you'll love.

To make your own flavored oil, add some preserved lemons or fresh herbs to plain olive oil.

1½ tablespoons hummus (no more than 3.5 grams of fat per 2 tablespoons)

1 tamari-seasoned organic brown rice cake or other seasoned brown rice cake (I used Lundberg Tamari with Seaweed Organic Rice Cakes)

8 very thin cucumber rounds

4 small or 2 large and very thin tomato slices

¼ teaspoon Meyer lemon-infused extra-virgin olive oil

Sea salt, to taste

Fresh ground black pepper, to taste

Spread the hummus evenly over the rice cake. Stack the cucumber and tomatoes on top of the hummus, starting with 4 cucumbers followed by 1 large or 2 small tomato slices. Then repeat the layers. Drizzle the oil over top and season with salt and pepper. Serve immediately.

Makes 1 serving

Per serving: 130 calories, 4 g protein, 21 g carbohydrates (3 g sugar), 4 g fat, <1 g saturated fat, 0 mg cholesterol, 4 g fiber, 169 mg sodium

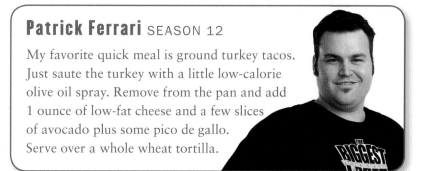

Patrick Ferrari SEASON 12

My favorite quick meal is ground turkey tacos. Just saute the turkey with a little low-calorie olive oil spray. Remove from the pan and add 1 ounce of low-fat cheese and a few slices of avocado plus some pico de gallo. Serve over a whole wheat tortilla.

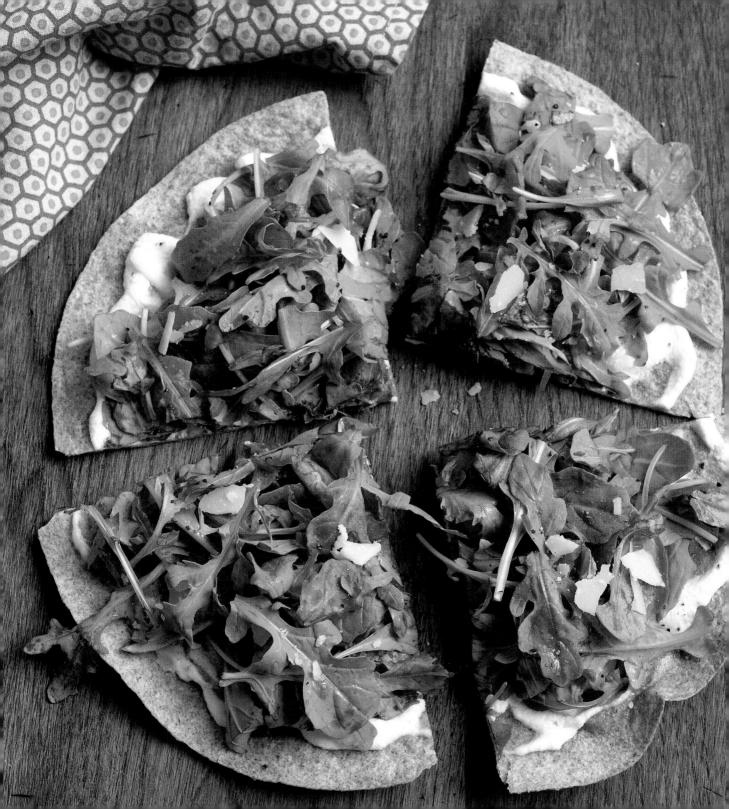

BLANCA ARUGULA PIZZA

A pizza like this could be called a salad pizza . . . or in this case, a white salad pizza. Regardless, it's an excellent way to satisfy a craving for an extra-thin and crispy pizza while also eating a substantial amount of greens.

It's really important that you do not use a flour tortilla that's artificially low carb in this recipe. They won't crisp properly, and they are often full of chemicals (and taste like it, too). I love French Meadow Bakery's Organic Sprouted Grain Tortillas—they are particularly tasty given how lean and clean they are.

---

1 (10") all-natural sprouted grain tortilla or other all-natural, low-fat whole grain tortilla (I used French Meadow Bakery Organic Sprouted Grain Tortillas)

¼ cup all-natural, fat-free ricotta cheese

¼ teaspoon garlic powder

Sea salt, to taste

Fresh ground black pepper, to taste

2 cups arugula leaves

1 teaspoon freshly squeezed lemon juice

½ teaspoon extra-virgin olive oil

¼ ounce shaved Parmesan or Romano cheese

Preheat the oven to 400°F.

Place the tortilla on a small nonstick baking sheet. Bake for 2 to 4 minutes per side, or until crisp. If air bubbles form during baking, poke the tortilla with a fork and then use a spatula or oven mitt to press the air out.

Meanwhile, in a small bowl, stir together the ricotta and garlic until well combined. Season with salt and pepper. Using the back of a spoon, spread the mixture evenly over the crisped tortilla, leaving about a ½" diameter bare. Bake the pizza for 3 to 5 minutes, or until the mixture is warmed through.

In a medium glass or plastic bowl, toss the arugula with the lemon juice and olive oil. Season with salt and pepper. Top the pizza evenly with the arugula, followed by the Parmesan. Serve immediately.

Makes 1 serving

Per serving: 263 calories, 18 g protein, 34 g carbohydrates (5 g sugar), 5 g fat, 2 g saturated fat, 17 mg cholesterol, 6 g fiber, 357 mg sodium

SUPER POWER SB&J ROLL

If PB&J still conjures happy memories of childhood, or if you make it for your kids, you'll love this updated, portable power snack version. I use sunflower seed butter instead of peanut butter for its anti-oxidant properties and because it's high in vitamin E, which is essential for cardiovascular health. Instead of the traditional grape or strawberry jam we all grew up on, I used an all-fruit super fruit spread. (If you have trouble finding it, try a pomegranate, acai, or even blueberry all-fruit spread.)

1 (10") all-natural sprouted grain tortilla or other (8") all-natural, low-fat whole grain tortilla (I used French Meadow Bakery Organic Sprouted Grain Tortillas)

1½ tablespoons all-natural, no sugar-added sunflower seed butter

1 tablespoon 100% fruit super fruit spread (I used Crofter's Organic SuperFruit Just Fruit Spread)

Place the tortilla on a clean, flat work surface. Spread it evenly with the sunflower seed butter to cover it completely. Then spread the fruit spread over all but 1" of one edge (the goal being to create a "glue" with the sunflower seed butter).

Starting at the edge opposite the one with no fruit spread, roll the tortilla. Serve immediately or wrap it in plastic wrap for a to-go snack.

Makes 1 serving

Per serving: 320 calories, 16 g protein, 41 g carbohydrates (10 g sugar), 10 g fat, 1 g saturated fat, 0 mg cholesterol, 8 g fiber, 219 mg sodium

>>> *TAKE IT TO GO!* >>>

This is such an easy snack to take on the road—perfect for kids' backpacks and grown-ups' lunch bags, too. Wrap the roll in plastic wrap or foil, or place it in a resealable plastic bag, and you're ready to head out the door. No refrigeration needed.

STEAMED SHRIMP WITH LEMON BUTTER FOR ONE

One night when I just couldn't find anything in the fridge to satisfy my hunger, I went tearing through the freezer and discovered some shrimp. I steamed it with the intention of making shrimp cocktail, but then realized I was out of cocktail sauce. Suddenly it occurred to me that I could treat the shrimp a bit like lobster—dip them in lemon butter. Obviously, traditional lobster butter is heavy on the butter and light on the lemon. Here I've reversed it for a healthy treat I enjoy often.

Save money by buying a big bag of frozen shrimp when it's on sale. Defrost it just before you're ready to eat it since it's super easy to thaw. Simply soak it in cold water for 5 to 10 minutes, and it'll be ready to cook.

---

5   ounces medium or large shrimp, peel on*

1   teaspoon natural whipped butter spread (I used Earth Balance Whipped Organic Buttery Spread)

1   tablespoon freshly squeezed lemon juice

Pour 1" of water in a shallow saucepan with a steamer insert. Place it over high heat and bring the water to a boil. Add the shrimp to the steamer in a single layer, if possible. Cook, covered, for 2 to 6 minutes, depending on the size, or until pink on the outsides and no longer translucent in the centers.

Meanwhile, in a small microwave-safe bowl, melt the butter. Add the lemon juice and stir until well combined.

Serve the shrimp immediately with the butter sauce for dipping.

Makes 1 serving

> Per serving: 151 calories, 23 g protein, 2 g carbohydrates (<1 g sugar), 5 g fat, 1 g saturated fat, 172 mg cholesterol, trace fiber, 201 mg sodium

*When buying shrimp, try to find some that have the peel on but are deveined. It will save time, yet you'll still get the added taste benefit of steaming them in the shell. If you buy the shrimp frozen, make sure they're defrosted before you start cooking. The measurement for this recipe is for 5 ounces of defrosted shrimp.

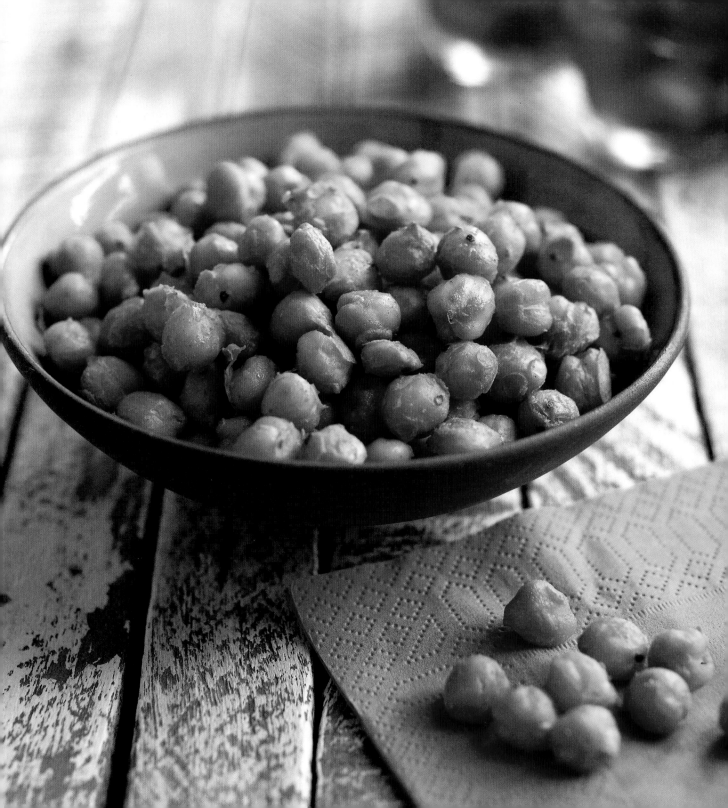

CRUNCHY CAJUN CHICKPEAS

These chickpeas are a great alternative when you're craving something salty and crunchy. Try them instead of corn nuts or potato chips for snacking. Or get extra creative and throw them in salads as a substitute for croutons, which tend to be full of empty calories.

Note that the nutritional information provided below is based on consuming only half of the salt, cayenne, black pepper, garlic powder, egg substitute, and flour called for in the recipe. That's because about half of it will be stuck inside the bowl or drip off onto the baking sheet. If you're watching your sodium intake carefully, be mindful that about half of it is actually dripping away.

Olive oil spray (propellant free)

1 tablespoon all-natural egg substitute

½ tablespoon whole grain oat flour

1 teaspoon paprika

¼ teaspoon salt

¼ teaspoon fresh ground black pepper

¼ teaspoon cayenne

⅛ teaspoon garlic powder

1 can (15 ounces) no-salt-added chickpeas, drained, rinsed and patted dry

Preheat the oven to 375°F. Mist a large nonstick baking sheet with the olive oil spray.

In a medium bowl, whisk the egg substitute, flour, paprika, salt, black pepper, cayenne, and garlic powder together until combined. Add the chickpeas and toss to coat. Place them on the prepared baking sheet in a single layer so they do not touch.

Bake for 15 minutes, then rotate the chickpeas with a spatula. Bake for 17 to 20 minutes longer, or until crispy and hot. Serve immediately.

Makes 2 (heaping ½ cup) servings

Per serving: 222 calories, 12 g protein, 39 g carbohydrates (2 g sugar), 2 g fat, trace saturated fat, 0 mg cholesterol, 8 g fiber, 210 mg sodium

Joe Mitchell SEASON 12

I love to spread a couple of Crispbread crackers with a little bit of goat cheese. I then throw one or two pieces of lean ham on top, and it's like a fast and healthy crispy sandwich.

BACON-WRAPPED GREEN BEAN BUNDLES

Let's face it: We Americans love our bacon. I recently even saw a maple-glazed doughnut with a slice of bacon on top—gasp! Hopefully Bob and Anna won't ever see that touch a contestant's lips.

Regardless, I've proven over and over that it's okay to have favorite foods and comfort foods. This recipe is no exception when it comes to bacon. This fun, easy appetizer is a perfect example of what you might consider making the next time a bacon craving strikes.

Olive oil spray (propellant free)

36 green beans, trimmed

1 teaspoon extra-virgin olive oil

¼ teaspoon fresh ground black pepper, or more to taste

6 slices 94% fat-free or leaner nitrate-free turkey bacon, cut in half crosswise

Preheat the oven to 400°F. Line a small baking sheet with nonstick foil. Lightly mist the foil with the olive oil spray.

In a small glass or plastic mixing bowl, toss the green beans with the oil and pepper.

Place a strip of bacon vertically on a cutting board. Lay 3 green beans horizontally across the end of the bacon closest to you. Roll the bacon tightly around the beans until you reach the opposite end of the bacon. Secure with a toothpick, if necessary, and place on the prepared baking sheet. Repeat the rolling 11 times with the remaining bacon and beans.

Bake for 8 to 10 minutes, or until the beans are crisp-tender and the bacon is lightly browned.

Makes 4 (3-bundle) servings

Per serving: 79 calories, 10 g protein, 4 g carbohydrates (2 g sugar), 3 g fat, trace saturated fat, 38 mg cholesterol, 2 g fiber, 300 mg sodium

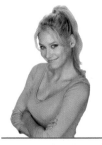

Biggest Loser Trainer Tip: Anna Kournikova

During the day I like to take a baggie with me that contains snacks like a slice of turkey wrapped around veggies or a small serving of almonds.

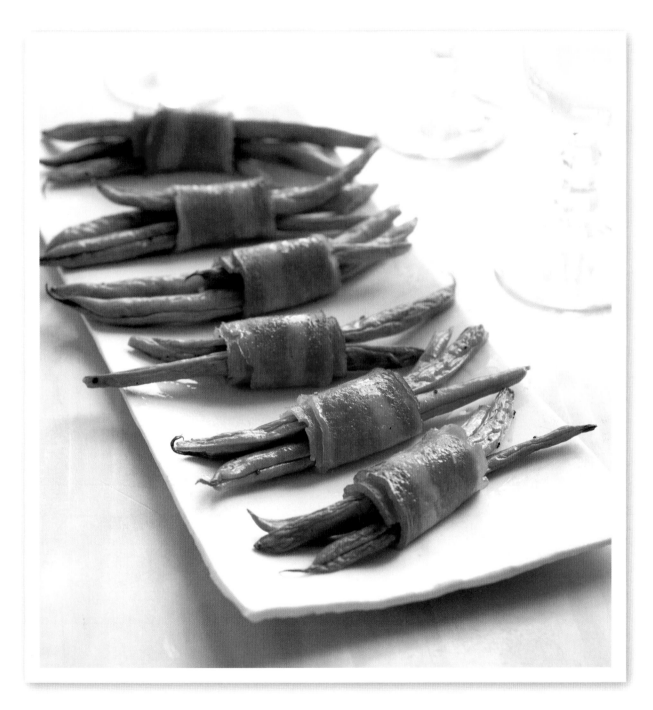

DOCTOR KRACKER TURKEY SNACKER

Crackers aren't just for cheese anymore. Many years ago, I fell in love with eating turkey on (healthy) crackers instead of bread. It's since caught on with many Biggest Loser contestants and even Biggest Loser fans.

Here's a quick snack that my whole team frequently enjoys. Feel free to put it on any cracker, though I particularly love the super-crispness of Doctor Kracker Flatbread Crackers. Plus, the pumpkin seed Cheddar variety, which is my favorite, has exactly 100 calories per (big) flatbread.

---

1 (about 25 grams) all-natural whole grain flatbread cracker (about 100 calories with at least 3 grams of fiber; I used Doctor Kracker Organic and Artisan-Baked Pumpkin Seed Cheddar Flatbreads)

1 tablespoon all-natural light herbed cheese spread (no more than 3.5 grams of fat per 2-tablespoon serving; I used Alouette Light Garlic and Herbs Soft Spreadable Cheese)

2 ounces very thinly sliced extra-lean, low-sodium, nitrate-free turkey (I used Presto Pesto Turkey Breast Roast, page 189)

Handful of watercress leaves

Place the cracker, seeds down, on a plate. Spread the cheese evenly over the entire cracker. Top it with the turkey, then the watercress. Serve immediately.

Makes 1 serving

> **Per serving:** 196 calories, 19 g protein, 12 g carbohydrates (1 g sugar), 8 g fat, 3 g saturated fat, 33 mg cholesterol, 4 g fiber, 278 mg sodium

MAKE A DIFFERENCE IN 20 MINUTES
The Lose Tube

You've heard it a million times—watching TV is not a good way to burn calories, and most people tend to overeat when they snack in front of the tube. But you don't have to give up TV to lose weight, just get active while you watch. The next time *The Biggest Loser* is on, jump rope for 20 minutes continuously while the contestants sweat their way through a challenge. You could burn a whopping 160 calories!

SOOO NOT CHICKEN NUGGETS

I often joke that my career has been a series of errors that often yielded great results. Though I went to culinary school, I never planned to be a chef, and a lot of my recipes are a result of my trying one thing and then happening upon something else in the process.

This recipe is a great example of that. Since deli turkey meat has so much sodium, I set out to make a grilled cheese and turkey with ground turkey instead of deli turkey. But, long story short, minus the cheese, I thought this dish tasted so similar to chicken nuggets that my friend's children might like it. So I made it for them one night, and now they beg their mom to make it all the time!

1 (8") all-natural, low-fat whole grain tortilla (I used Rudi's Organic Bakery Whole Spelt Tortillas)

4 ounces ground turkey breast

1 tablespoon all-natural ketchup (preferably agave- or honey-sweetened and low in salt), or more to taste

Preheat the oven 450°F.

Lay the tortilla on a medium baking sheet. Press the turkey in a thin, even layer to cover all but the outer $\frac{1}{2}$"-diameter of the tortilla. Fold the tortilla in half and press to flatten it slightly. Bake for 3 minutes. Carefully flip the tortilla and bake for 3 to 5 minutes longer, or until the tortilla is lightly crisped and the turkey is no longer pink inside.

Using kitchen shears for ease, cut it into 4 wedges. Serve immediately with ketchup on the side for dipping.

Makes 1 serving

Per serving: **280 calories, 33 g protein, 32 g carbohydrates (2 g sugar), 5 g fat, 1 g saturated fat, 45 mg cholesterol, 2 g fiber, 265 mg sodium**

Hannah Curlee SEASON 11 FINALIST

When I get a chocolate craving, I snack on Greek yogurt mixed with cocoa powder, Truvía, and vanilla. It's a little more than 100 calories, and it tastes like chocolate pudding!

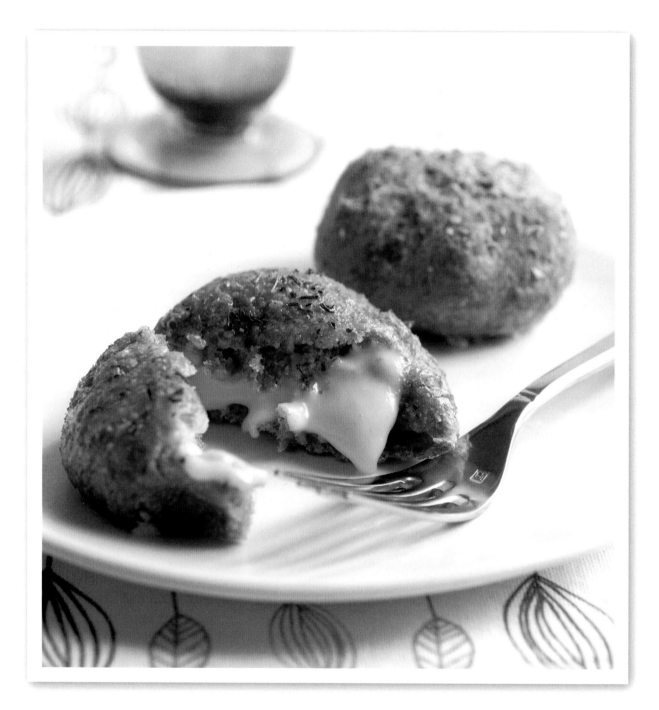

BAKED BABYBELS

These yummy appetizers are inspired by one of my favorite party foods: baked brie. Make them without the garlic herb blend, and they are cheesy, gooey deliciousness. Make them with the seasoning, and they feel like they belong in a pizzeria. Either way (or both!), you're sure to enjoy this comforting snack.

Most store-bought wheat dough is not excessively sticky, so you don't need flour to press it out. I like to keep the calories to a minimum, so I don't use the flour. If you find that the dough you've purchased is too sticky to work with, however, try using as little whole wheat pastry flour as possible to dust your work surface and your hands.

Olive oil spray (propellant free)

3 **ounces all-natural whole wheat pizza dough (no more than 3 grams of fat per 2-ounce serving)**

½ **teaspoon salt-free garlic seasoning blend (I used The Spice Hunter Salt Free Garlic Herb Bread Blend)**

2 **rounds (21 grams each) Laughing Cow Mini Babybel Light, sliced in half to create two rounds (not 2 half circles)**

Preheat the oven 450°F. Place a sheet of nonstick foil on a small baking sheet. Lightly mist the foil with the olive oil spray.

Shape the pizza dough into 4 balls that weigh ¾ ounce each. On a clean work surface, using your hands, flatten each until each is just large enough to completely enclose a cheese round. Sprinkle ⅛ teaspoon of the seasoning on each dough circle. Place one cheese circle in the center of each of the dough circles.

Carefully stretch the bare dough up and to the center so that the edges connect on top and the cheese is sealed inside. Make sure the bottom isn't any thinner than the rest of the dough, and be careful not to create any holes in the dough. Place them side by side, sealed sides up, on the prepared baking sheet, making sure they do not touch. Sprinkle the top of each with a few extra flecks of the seasoning to add color, if desired.

Bake for 5 to 7 minutes, watching them carefully during the last few minutes, or until the dough is cooked. You want to remove them from the oven before the cheese oozes out. Serve immediately.

Makes 2 (2-ball) servings

Per serving: 148 calories, 9 g protein, 18 g carbohydrates (<1 g sugar), 4 g fat, 2 g saturated fat, 15 mg cholesterol, 2 g fiber, 339 mg sodium

HONEY NUT APPLE BUTTER RICE CAKES

Yes, this recipe is no-brainer easy. And that's what people constantly ask me for: easy snacks that they can throw together in a minute. Though I certainly wouldn't want to give you a whole cookbook of simple ideas like this one, I wanted to include this particular recipe because it's 100 calories of pure yumminess!

1   honey nut (or other sweet variety) brown rice cake (I used Lundberg Honey Nut Rice Cakes)

1   tablespoon no-sugar-added 100% fruit apple butter (I used Kozlowski Farms 100% Fruit Sweetened Apple Butter)

Place the rice cake on a flat work surface. Spread the apple butter on one side of the rice cake. Serve immediately.

Makes 1 serving

Per serving: **100 calories, 1 g protein, 24 g carbohydrates (9 g sugar), <1 g fat, 0 g saturated fat, 0 mg cholesterol, 1 g fiber, 35 mg sodium**

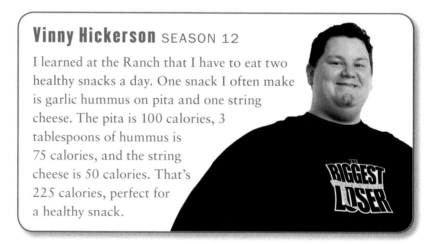

Vinny Hickerson SEASON 12

I learned at the Ranch that I have to eat two healthy snacks a day. One snack I often make is garlic hummus on pita and one string cheese. The pita is 100 calories, 3 tablespoons of hummus is 75 calories, and the string cheese is 50 calories. That's 225 calories, perfect for a healthy snack.

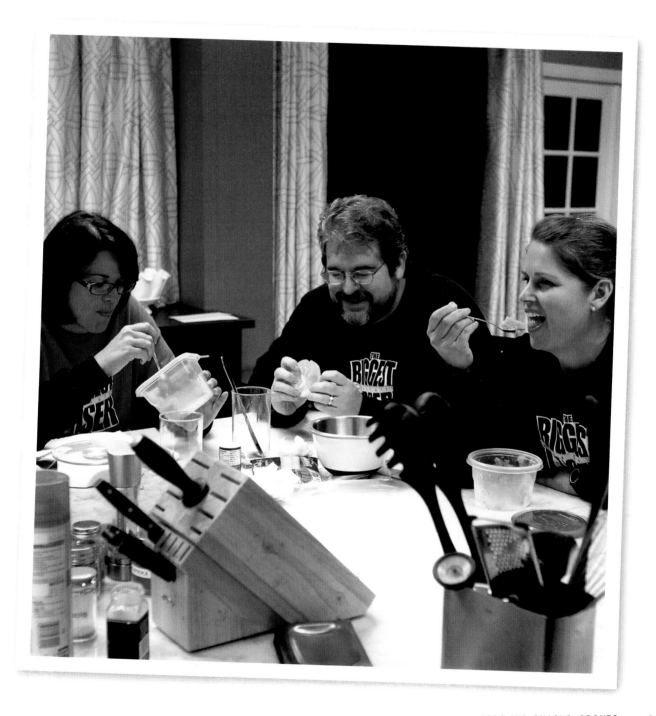

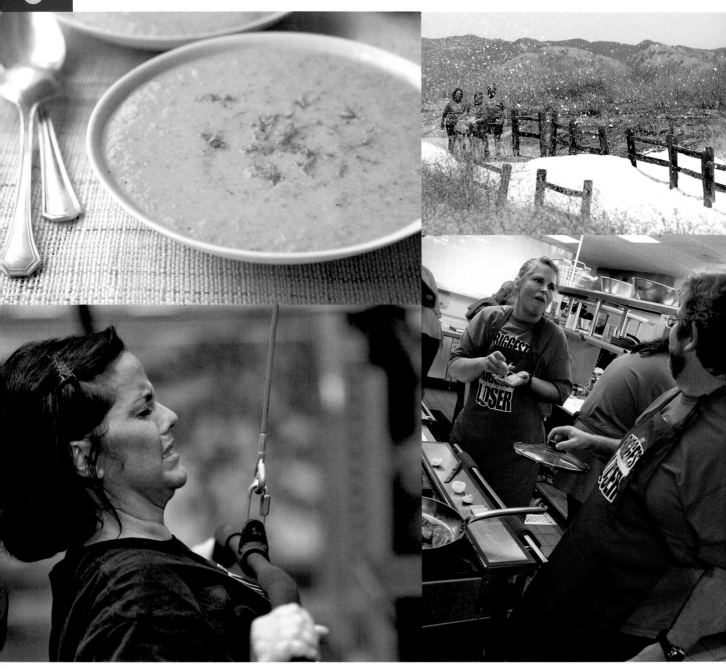

5

Speedy Soups and Sandwiches

Burgers, wraps, and sandwiches fulfill a certain comfort-food craving. When you really want to sink your teeth into something satisfying, a juicy burger or a tasty sandwich or wrap just hits the spot.

Season 12's Jessica Limpert says she's a fan of making healthy sandwiches using whole wheat pita bread. "I just slice it open and fill it with 1 cup of mixed lettuce, some yellow mustard, sliced onions, jalapeños, green and red peppers, and about 2 ounces of roast beef or turkey breast. It's very filling!"

As Chef Devin knows all too well, a lot of *Biggest Loser* contestants come to the Ranch with a burger-a-day habit. She developed her patriotically named Red, White, and Blue Burger (page 115) to help them satisfy their fast-food craving in a much more nutritious way.

"So many of the contestants have a long history with fast food, and burgers are one of the things they miss the most when they come to the Ranch," she says. "I love developing recipes like this one, which I know will satisfy that 'must-have' craving but won't undermine their weight-loss efforts."

Soups can add a variety of flavors and textures to your meal without a lot of calories. While some heartier soups are often an entrée by themselves, the light, low-calorie soups in this chapter give you endless options. You can pair them with a salad, a side, or half a sandwich for a full meal. Try the Cold Cucumber Soup (page 126) with half of the Herb Turkey Sandwich (page 123), or the Simple Strawberry Soup (page 128) with a Watermelon Feta Salad (page 137).

Some studies even suggest that eating soup as part of a meal can actually help you lose weight. Researchers at Penn State University found that people who ate a serving of low-calorie soup before their entrée reduced their total calorie intake for the meal by one-fifth compared to participants who ate the entrée alone. If you're eating a 300-calorie meal, that's a savings of 60 calories!

And here's another secret about soups: They're a great way to get kids to eat their fruits and veggies. A lot of kids don't like the texture of fruits and vegetables, but when you add some veggies to the blender and create a spoonable soup, they won't know that there's "healthy stuff" lurking in their bowl. Serve a simple carrot or broccoli soup with whole wheat bread or crackers for dipping, and they'll have a ball playing with their food.

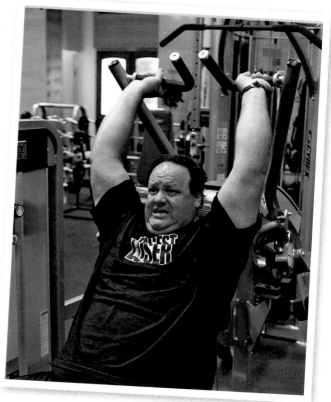

Dan Evans SEASON 11

My favorite dish is a very simple BLT that uses thin wheat bread, turkey bacon (I swear it tastes just like regular bacon), and lettuce. When I really splurge, I add a dab of low-calorie cream cheese instead of low-fat mayo. It's just something I invented with what was in the Ranch kitchen, and it's only about 150 calories!

RED, WHITE, AND BLUE BURGER

I always say that a burger isn't a burger unless you require a napkin to eat it! This burger certainly meets that standard. Just be sure not to press on the patties with the back of a spatula while they're cooking. A lot of people think that doing so removes excess fat, but particularly when you're using a lean cut of beef, all you're doing is removing moisture from the meat. When properly cooked, a burger should be nice and juicy—and the toppings add to the drip factor. Yum!

You can save even more time by buying preshaped burger patties, if you can find them.

---

1 teaspoon salt-free Cajun or Creole seasoning (I used The Spice Hunter Salt Free Cajun Creole Seasoning Blend)

4 ounces 96% lean ground beef patty

1 all-natural whole grain or whole wheat English muffin (I used Rudi's Organic Bakery Whole Grain Wheat English Muffins), split*

½ tablespoon all-natural light sandwich spread (I used Spectrum Naturals Light Canola Mayo)

1 tablespoon all-natural, reduced-fat blue cheese crumbles

A few baby mixed green lettuce leaves, or more to taste

1 large tomato slice

Preheat a grill to high.

Sprinkle the seasoning evenly over the patty. Grill the beef for 1 to 2 minutes per side, for medium rare, or until desired doneness is reached. Toast the English muffin halves, cut sides down, on an upper grill rack or away from the direct flame, for 30 seconds to 1 minute.

Place the muffin bottom, toasted side up, on a serving plate. Evenly spread it with sandwich spread. Add the burger, then the blue cheese crumbles, lettuce, and the tomato. Flip the second muffin half on top. Serve immediately.

Makes 1 serving

> **Per serving:** 312 calories, 30 g protein, 28 g carbohydrates (3 g sugar), 9 g fat, 3 g saturated fat, 64 mg cholesterol, 4 g fiber, 450 mg sodium

*You can certainly use an all-natural, low-fat whole grain 3½"-diameter hamburger bun. However, I've found that these are often dry and take away from the hamburger experience. Instead, I opt for the English muffin, which, in the case of Rudi's, is tastier than any "healthy" hamburger bun I've been able to find.

CAPRESE BURGER

I know that a lot of people prolong the life of fresh herbs by finely chopping them, packing them into ice cube trays, then adding just enough water to freeze them. I've never loved that technique (though I know many folks do). What I do love, however, are the little blocks of herbs that are popping up in grocery stores everywhere. The most common brand in my area is Dorot. I especially like to use the basil cubes to create quick and easy pestos with virtually no effort.

1 tablespoon all-natural light sandwich spread (I used Spectrum Naturals Light Canola Mayo)

1 cube (3.5 grams) frozen basil, thawed (I used Dorot All-Natural Chopped Basil)

4 ounces 96% lean ground beef patty

Salt, to taste

½ ounce very thinly sliced almond mozzarella cheese (I use Lisanatti)

1 all-natural whole grain or whole wheat English muffin (I used Rudi's Organic Bakery Whole Grain Wheat English Muffin), split

Small handful of arugula leaves

¼"-thick large tomato slice

Preheat a grill to high.

In a small bowl, stir the sandwich spread and basil until combined.

Season both sides of the patty with salt. Grill for 1 to 2 minutes per side for medium rare, or until desired doneness is reached. About 1 minute before the burger is done, add the cheese and melt for 1 minute.

Meanwhile, place the muffin halves on the grill away from the direct flame to warm them.

Place the muffin bottom, cut side up, on a serving plate. Top it with the arugula, the burger, and then the tomato. Spread the pesto mayo evenly over the inside of the top of the English muffin and place it atop the burger. Serve immediately.

Makes 1 serving

Per serving: 333 calories, 31 g protein, 27 g carbohydrates (3 g sugar), 10 g fat, 2 g saturated fat, 60 mg cholesterol, 4 g fiber, 513 mg sodium

Ken Andrews SEASON 11

One of my favorite lunches now is a Greek pita sandwich. I use turkey, lettuce, a few olives, mushrooms, and low-fat feta. Mix it all up and stuff it in the pita.

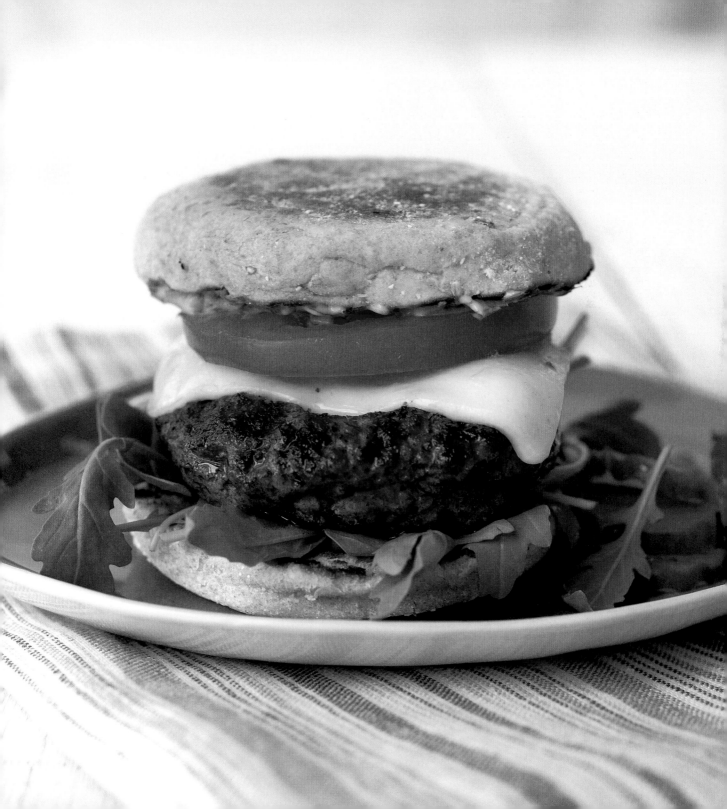

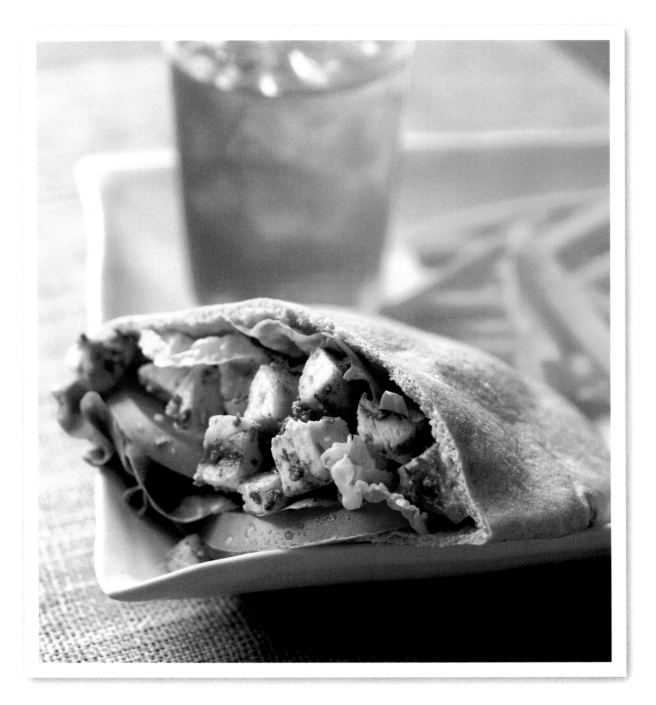

OLIVE CHICKEN SALAD PITA

Olives are a good source of vitamin E and contain beneficial fats. Thus they can make a great spread or healthy addition to a dressing or salad—as long as they're used in moderation. Here, instead of mixing chicken with mayonnaise, I mix it with an olive tapenade. Not only do you get a punch of flavor, it makes a yummy, simple chicken salad to throw into a pita.

4 ounces lean natural grilled chicken breast or Essential Grilled Chicken (page xxii), cut into small (about ⅓") cubes

1 tablespoon all-natural olive tapenade

1 (7"-diameter) all-natural whole wheat pita pocket (look for one with less than 2 grams of fat and 240 milligrams of sodium plus a few grams of fiber per pita)

Handful of baby mixed green lettuce leaves, or more to taste

2 (⅛"-thick) large tomato slices

In a small mixing bowl, toss the chicken with the tapenade.

Cut one-third of the pita circle off and reserve it for another recipe.

Stuff the remaining pita pocket with the chicken. Add the lettuce and tomatoes. Serve immediately, or wrap and refrigerate it until ready to enjoy.

Makes 1 serving

Per serving: **297 calories, 31 g protein, 23 g carbohydrates (< 1 g sugar), 9 g fat, <1 g saturated fat, 66 mg cholesterol, 5 g fiber, 452 mg sodium**

>>> TAKE IT TO GO! >>>

Pack the chicken salad in a resealable plastic container, and lay the tomato and lettuce flat on top of it. Pop the pita into a resealable plastic bag and you're ready to head out the door. Just be sure to keep the salad on ice or in a refrigerator until you're ready to assemble and enjoy.

CURRY IN A HURRY POCKET

This recipe is a great way to use the leftover pork from Curry-Rubbed Pork Tenderloin with Peach Chutney (page 177)—it's just as delicious in a sandwich as it is as an entrée. The broccoli and raita in the slaw add crunch and creaminess to the mildly spicy flavor of the tenderloin. If you want to add more raita to the pocket to make it even drippier, that's totally fine. Each tablespoon of the raita I found has only 12 calories and 1 gram of fat.

1 (7"-diameter) all-natural whole wheat pita pocket (look for one with less than 2 grams of fat and 240 milligrams of sodium per pita)

4 ounces Curry-Rubbed Pork Tenderloin (page 177), sliced very thin

1 cup Super Simple Slaw (page 148)

Cut one-third of the pita from the pita circle. Reserve it for another recipe.

Stuff the remaining pita pocket evenly with the pork (omitting the chutney), then the slaw. Serve immediately, or wrap and refrigerate it until ready to enjoy.

Makes 1 serving

Per serving: 273 calories, 30 g protein, 26 g carbohydrates (<1 g sugar), 6 g fat, 2 g saturated fat, 75 mg cholesterol, 5 g fiber, 362 mg sodium

MAKE A DIFFERENCE IN 20 MINUTES
Bored Meetings

Sometimes work can seem like one never-ending meeting. All of that sitting inevitably leads to coffee breaks, which inevitably add up to extra calories. Instead of heading to Starbucks the next time 4 o'clock rolls around, grab a colleague and go for a brisk 20-minute walk. You can even hold a walking meeting. Not only will you get some fresh air and sunshine, you can also burn about 105 calories.

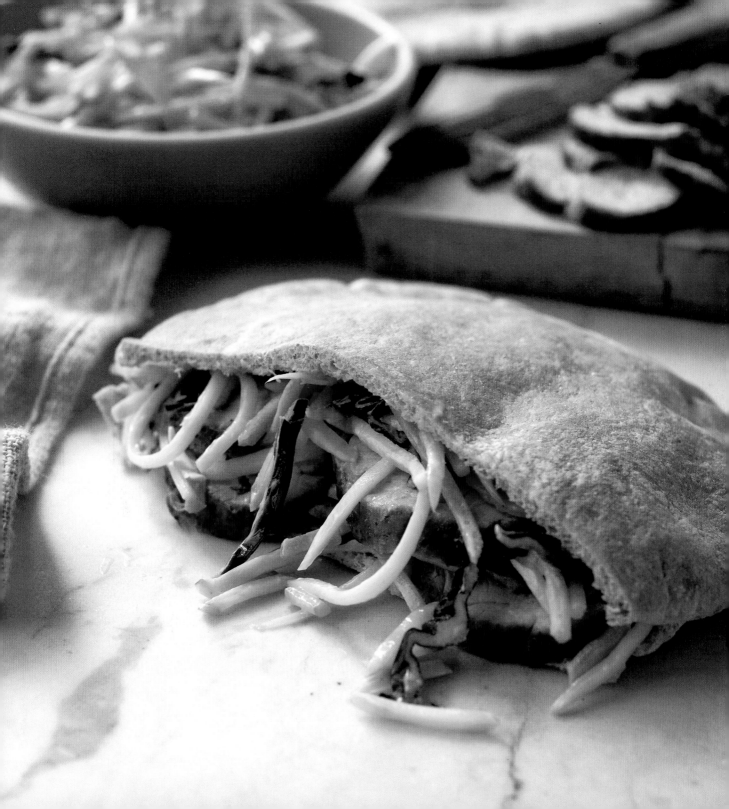

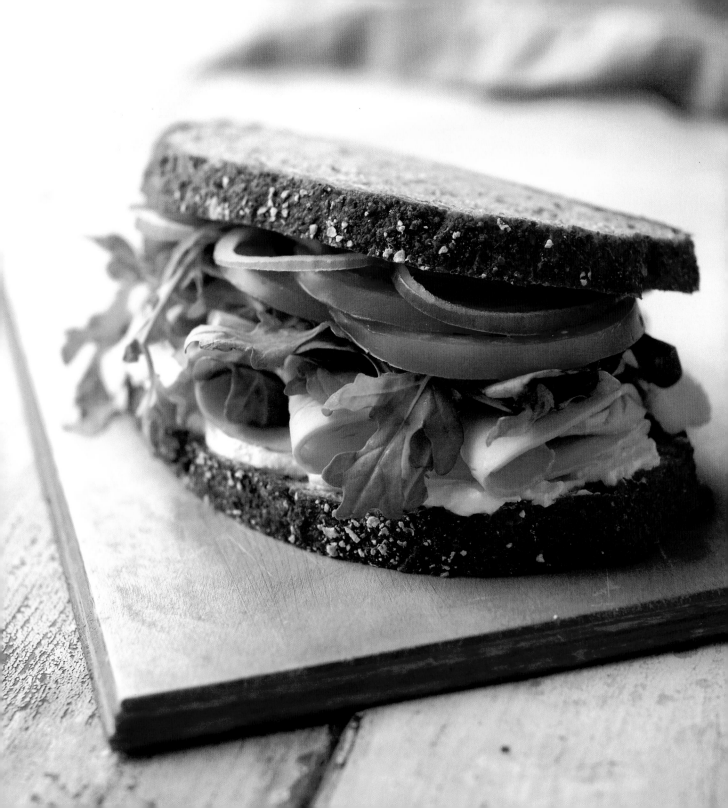

HERB TURKEY SANDWICH

Healthy breads tend to taste better when warmed, so I recommend you warm or toast the bread if you are not making this sandwich to go.

I use arugula leaves in this recipe and throughout the book because they add flavor and have more nutritional content than lighter-colored lettuces like iceberg. If you find the taste of arugula too bitter, you can substitute other dark greens, such as pepper watercress or baby spinach leaves.

2 slices all-natural whole grain sourdough bread (no more than 70 calories per slice; I used Julian Bakery Amazing Sourdough)

2 tablespoons herb and garlic goat cheese spread (choose one with no more than 50 calories and 3.5 grams of fat per 2-tablespoon serving; I used Chavrie with Basil and Roasted Garlic Goat's Milk Cheese spread)

4 ounces very thinly sliced low-sodium, nitrate-free, lean roasted turkey breast (I used Presto Pesto Turkey Breast Roast, see page 189)

Handful of arugula leaves

4 (⅛"-thick) medium tomato slices

A few very thin slices red onion, or more to taste

Place 1 slice of bread on a plate. Spread evenly with the cheese spread and pile the turkey evenly on top of it. Top the turkey with the arugula, tomatoes, and onions. Top that with the second slice of bread. Serve immediately, or wrap and refrigerate it until ready to enjoy.

Makes 1 serving

Per serving: 323 calories, 41 g protein, 25 g carbohydrates (2 g sugar), 7 g fat, 3 g saturated fat, 65 mg cholesterol, 13 g fiber, 518 mg sodium

Elizabeth Ruiz SEASON 10

I wasn't always a lettuce person, but I'm becoming one. You can make a sandwich using romaine lettuce leaves instead of bread. Pile on a few slices of roast beef, add onions and cilantro—it's awesome!

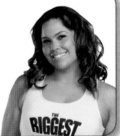

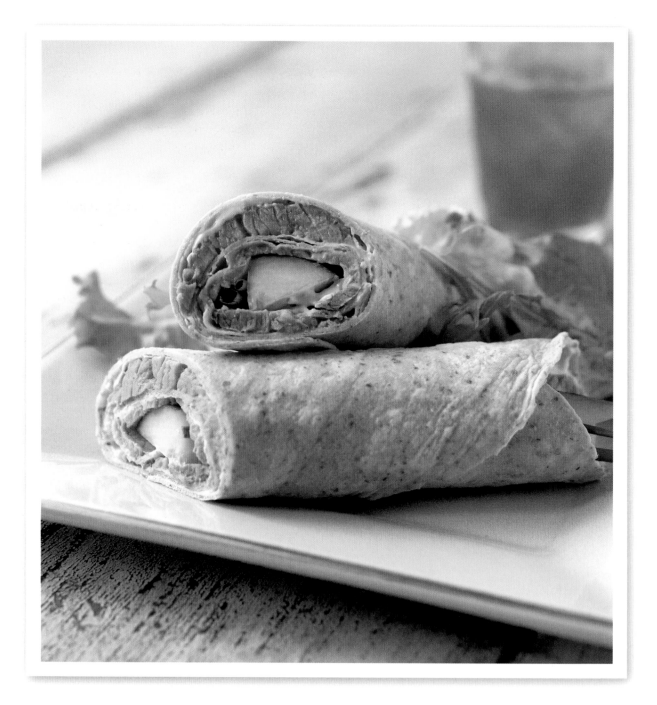

RBC ROLL

I call this version of a roast beef sandwich an RBC Roll because when you cut it into small pieces, it resembles a sushi roll—which makes it a great option for lunch, snacking, or serving as an hors d'oeuvre. The cucumber is intended to resemble a wedge of cucumber you'd see in a sushi roll. To cut it, just trim the ends, then cut it in half lengthwise. Cut those halves in half again. If the cucumber was thick, halve them one more time. Reserve any leftovers for munching or for another recipe.

1 (10") all-natural sprouted grain tortilla or other (8") all-natural, low-fat whole grain tortilla (I used French Meadow Bakery Organic Sprouted Grain Tortillas)

1 tablespoon all-natural light herbed cheese spread (I used Alouette Light Garlic and Herbs Soft Spreadable Cheese)

3 ounces very thinly sliced nitrate-free, low-sodium lean roast beef (I used Chili-Rubbed London Broil, see page 166)

Wedge of cucumber the length of the tortilla

3 chives, cut to 7" if longer than that

Place the tortilla on a cutting board. Spread the cheese spread evenly over it. Cover two-thirds of the cheese with the roast beef. Place the cucumber and chives together on the edge with the meat, opposite the cheese-only portion. Roll the tortilla tightly, starting by wrapping it around the cucumber and chives until you reach the other side. Serve immediately or store it in a resealable plastic bag and refrigerate until ready to eat.

Makes 1 serving

Per serving: 270 calories, 28 g protein, 29 g carbohydrates (3 g sugar), 6 g fat, 3 g saturated fat, 44 mg cholesterol, 6 g fiber, 391 mg sodium

Bonnie Griffin SEASON 12

Don't *ever* go to the store without a shopping list. Always plan ahead. That way you'll be less tempted to buy junk or processed foods impulsively.

COLD CUCUMBER SOUP

You can use traditional cucumbers—though you will want about 5 large ones instead of 3 medium English (or hothouse) cucumbers—to make this yummy, refreshing soup. Just be sure to seed them. English cucumbers don't need to be seeded, so they keep the recipe super quick.

If you're new to seeding cucumbers, just cut them in half lengthwise and then use a teaspoon (the kind you eat with, not the kind you measure ingredients with) to scrape the center of the cucumbers from one end to the other to remove the seeds.

3 medium English cucumbers, peeled and cut into large pieces

4 medium cloves garlic, peeled and trimmed

1 cup fat-free Greek yogurt

⅔ cup low-fat sour cream

1 tablespoon all-natural Dijon mustard, preferably with no added sugar

2 tablespoons dill leaves, or more to taste

Sea salt, to taste

1 medium (regular) cucumber, seeded and cut into ½" pieces

Add the English cucumber pieces and garlic to the bowl of a food processor fitted with a chopping blade. Pulse the mixture so the veggies are finely chopped. Add the yogurt, sour cream, mustard, dill, and salt and pulse the mixture until it is the consistency of soup. Pour the mixture into a large glass or plastic mixing bowl. Stir in the ½" cucumber pieces and serve immediately.

Makes 4 servings (about 7½ cups)

Per serving: 135 calories, 10 g protein, 17 g carbohydrates (11 g sugar), 3 g fat, 1 g saturated fat, 13 mg cholesterol, 4 g fiber, 103 mg sodium

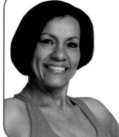

Miggy Cancel SEASON 9

I like to combine different kinds of beans like white, red, and black. Add cucumber and tomatoes, some fresh cilantro, and olive oil. Let the salad marinate for a few hours. It's a high source of protein and a convenient meal!

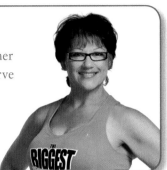

Patti Anderson SEASON 9

I've been cooking healthy even at dinner parties. We love to entertain, and I serve a grilled portobello cap topped with low-fat marinara sauce and low-fat mozzarella cheese. It's delicious! No one misses the calories.

Biggest Loser Club Expert Tip: Greg Hottinger, RD

Making your own soups is super easy and better tasting than most canned varieties, plus you avoid all the sodium they contain. All you need to do is chop up carrots, celery, onion, a bell pepper, if you like, and garlic, and add to a large pot. Then add water or low-sodium broth and cook.

Add seasonings like oregano or rosemary or whatever you like—the possibilities are really endless. Here's a basic quick-and-easy recipe. Feel free to alter as desired.

½ small onion, chopped

2 cloves garlic, chopped

Ginger, minced

1 medium white potato, chopped into small pieces

2 large carrots, chopped

2 stalks celery, chopped

½ teaspoon salt

6 cups water

Fresh ground black pepper or white pepper, to taste

In a soup pot, combine all of the ingredients. Bring to a soft boil for 2 to 3 minutes, then reduce the heat to medium. Simmer, covered, for 15 minutes, or until all of the vegetables are tender.

That's it. You can add some chicken or white fish if you want protein in this soup. It will keep you warm and satisfied!

SIMPLE STRAWBERRY SOUP

This is a very light, refreshing, tart soup that makes a perfect lunch when paired with half a sandwich or a salad. Strawberries can vary in sweetness, depending on their ripeness and the time of year, so taste your soup before serving. If it is too tart, add more honey, just a bit at a time, until it is sweet enough for you.

2½ cups frozen strawberries, thawed

¼ cup freshly squeezed lime juice

½ cup fat-free, preferably fruit juice–sweetened vanilla yogurt

2 teaspoons honey, or to taste

Lime zest, to taste

Add the strawberries, lime juice, yogurt, and honey to the bowl of a food processor fitted with a chopping blade. Process until the mixture is smooth. Divide the soup among 2 bowls and garnish with lime zest. Serve immediately.

Makes 2 (1-cup) servings

Per serving: **134 calories, 4 g protein, 32 g carbohydrates (20 g sugar), trace fat, trace saturated fat, 0 mg cholesterol, 4 g fiber, 35 mg sodium**

>>> TAKE IT TO GO! >>>

This pretty soup is likely to be the envy of your coworkers if you show up with a resealable plastic container of it. Just be sure to store it in a refrigerator or on ice before you flaunt it. And don't forget to pack a spoon!

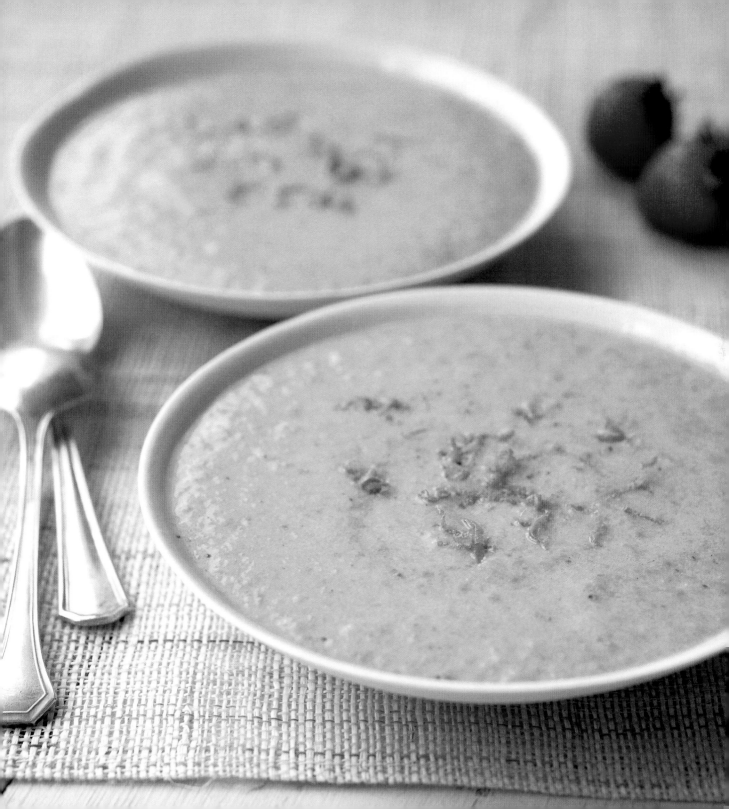

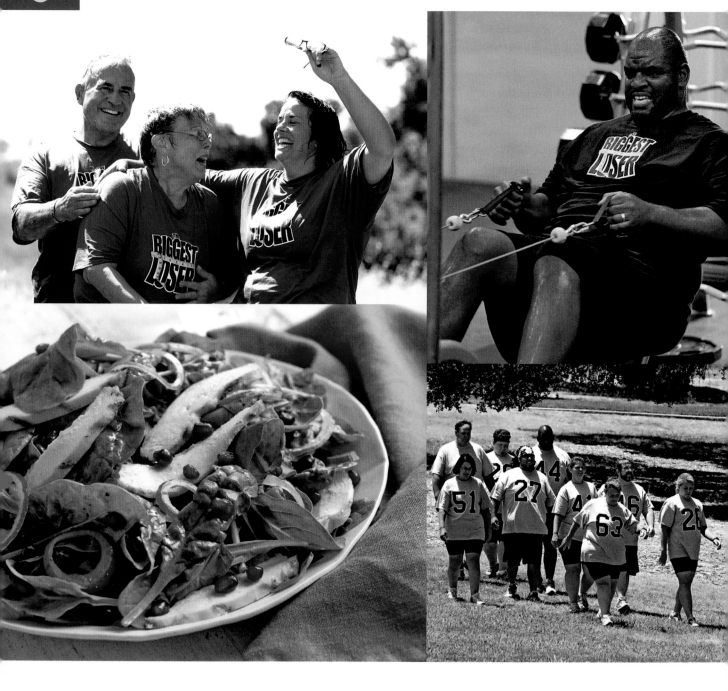

6

Throw-Together Salads and Sides

As adults, we all know that we should eat plenty of fruits and vegetables. Fresh produce is not only filling, low in calories, and high in fiber, it also offers a wide range of health benefits, including vitamins and minerals that promote cardiovascular health, decrease the risk of developing diseases like cancer and type 2 diabetes, and boost our immune function.

That's a lot of upside for simply eating your fruits and veggies. So how many servings do you eat a day?

If you're like most Americans, not many at all. In 2010 the US Centers for Disease Control and Prevention (CDC) published a study of fruit and vegetable consumption among adults by state. Researchers found that 32.5 percent of American adults, on average, consumed fruit two or more times a day (with Oklahoma winning the unfortunate title of the lowest fruit-consuming population). The percentage of adults who consumed vegetables three or more times a day was even lower: a measly 26.3 percent (with South Dakota earning the infamous distinction of lowest veggie-consuming population).

On *The Biggest Loser* eating plan, you should aim for a minimum of 4 cups daily of a variety of fruits and nonstarchy vegetables. If fresh fruits and vegetables aren't available, are out of season, or are too expensive, it's fine to substitute frozen fruits and veggies to meet your daily requirements. As long as they don't contain any added sugar or sodium, they can be just as nutritious as fresh.

"Stock up on frozen veggies. They're quick and easy if you don't have fresh vegetables on hand for a particular recipe," advises Bob Harper. "We keep them in the *Biggest Loser* kitchen on the Ranch." Season 12's Bonnie Griffin says she buys extra fruit when it's in season and then cuts it up and freezes it so that she can make delicious fruit smoothies any time of the year.

One great strategy for fitting fruits and veggies into your day is to have a salad for one meal, either lunch or dinner. And if you're one of those people who thinks that salads are bland, boring, or just not filling, we have a feeling that after you try Chef Devin's tasty Pomegranate Spinach Salad (page 140) or her satisfying Chinese Dumpling Salad (page 134), you'll reconsider.

Another great strategy for getting your daily dose is to make sure that vegetables occupy significant real estate on your dinner plate. And no, that doesn't mean you have to eat steamed broccoli every day—and it also doesn't mean that french fries count as a vegetable. Many contestants arrive at the Ranch self-proclaimed veggie haters, but once they try out a variety of vegetables, they find new favorite foods.

Season 9's Darrell Hough admits, "I'd never eaten an eggplant before coming to the Ranch. I thought it would be purple inside! Now I grill them and put them on sandwiches. I love it. They have an earthy, delicious flavor."

With mouthwatering options like "Fried" Mushroom Parmesan Bake (page 150), Sesame Roasted Asparagus (page 153), and Gazpacho Quinoa (page 142), there's no excuse to skip your veggies!

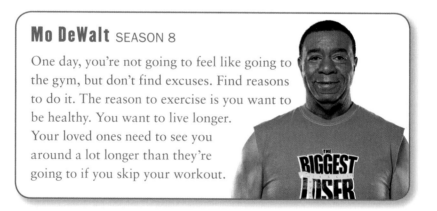

Mo DeWalt SEASON 8

One day, you're not going to feel like going to the gym, but don't find excuses. Find reasons to do it. The reason to exercise is you want to be healthy. You want to live longer. Your loved ones need to see you around a lot longer than they're going to if you skip your workout.

LOBSTER SLAW SALAD

If you've ever had lobster tacos, this recipe may seem familiar. Lobster tacos often contain a creamy lemon sauce, cabbage, and plenty of fresh salsa. Here, I combined those ingredients, minus the tortillas, into a yummy throw-together salad.

If you're not familiar with them, langostinos are small rock lobsters. Look for them in the freezer section of your grocery store. They're generally precooked, so all you have to do is defrost them, making this a super-easy weeknight dinner.

3 cups shredded cabbage

1 cup drained fresh (refrigerated) salsa

1 tablespoon all-natural light lemon-mayonnaise (no more than 40 calories and 4 grams of fat per tablespoon; I used The Ojai Cook Lemonaise Light)

1 tablespoon freshly squeezed lemon juice

¼ teaspoon salt-free fajita or Southwest seasoning

4 ounces langostinos,* thawed

In a large bowl, toss the cabbage, salsa, lemon-mayonnaise, lemon juice, and seasoning until well combined. Top it with the langostinos. Serve immediately.

Makes 1 serving

Per serving: 234 calories, 26 g protein, 24 g carbohydrates (7 g sugar), 5 g fat, <1 g saturated fat, 110 mg cholesterol, 8 g fiber, 506 mg sodium

If you can't find langostinos, you can always substitute an equal amount of steamed and chilled shrimp instead.

Amanda Arlauskas SEASON 8

When I used to watch TV, I would snack way too much on horrible foods. I would take a box of cereal and a gallon of milk, and keep refilling my bowl until I was full. Now, I love munching on baby carrots and hummus as a healthier alternative.

CHINESE DUMPLING SALAD

Here's a new take on a Chinese chicken salad. It allows you to enjoy chilled steamed pot stickers as part of the salad, to give it a hearty feel. Though there are a number of ingredients in this salad, it's still very simple to assemble and comes together in minutes.

---

3 preservative-free, low-fat whole wheat chicken pot stickers (about 190 calories and 1.5 grams of fat per 5-piece serving)*

2½ cups loosely packed mixed baby greens

2 cups shredded classic coleslaw mix

2 whole small scallions, trimmed and finely chopped

3 tablespoons shelled edamame (soybeans), thawed if frozen

¼ cup mung bean sprouts

2 tablespoons agave-sweetened or honey-sweetened all-natural Chinese dressing (make sure it's relatively low in fat, calories, and sodium; I used Follow Your Heart Organics Miso Ginger Salad Dressing)

3 ounces sliced Essential Grilled Chicken (page xxii), or other preservative-free lean grilled chicken

Place a steamer rack in a large pan or pot with a lid. Add water until it reaches just below the rack. Place the pan or pot over high heat and bring it to a boil. Add the pot stickers and steam, covered, for 4 to 6 minutes, or until they are hot through.

Meanwhile, in a medium mixing bowl, toss the greens, coleslaw mix, scallions, edamame, sprouts, and dressing. Mound the mixture on a serving plate and top it with the pot stickers and chicken.

Makes 1 serving

Per serving: **398 calories, 34 g protein, 43 g carbohydrates (12 g sugar), 14 g fat, 1 g saturated fat, 58 mg cholesterol, 9 g fiber, 670 mg sodium**

Look for pot stickers in the freezer section of the grocery store. And note that the front of the bag may not say "whole wheat" or "low-fat," even if they are. Be sure to read the nutrition label.

Aaron Thompkins SEASON 10

For a quick and easy supper salad, I toss together a bag of spring mix greens, a few strips of turkey bacon, boiled egg whites, and cherry tomatoes. It's like a chef's salad but way healthier.

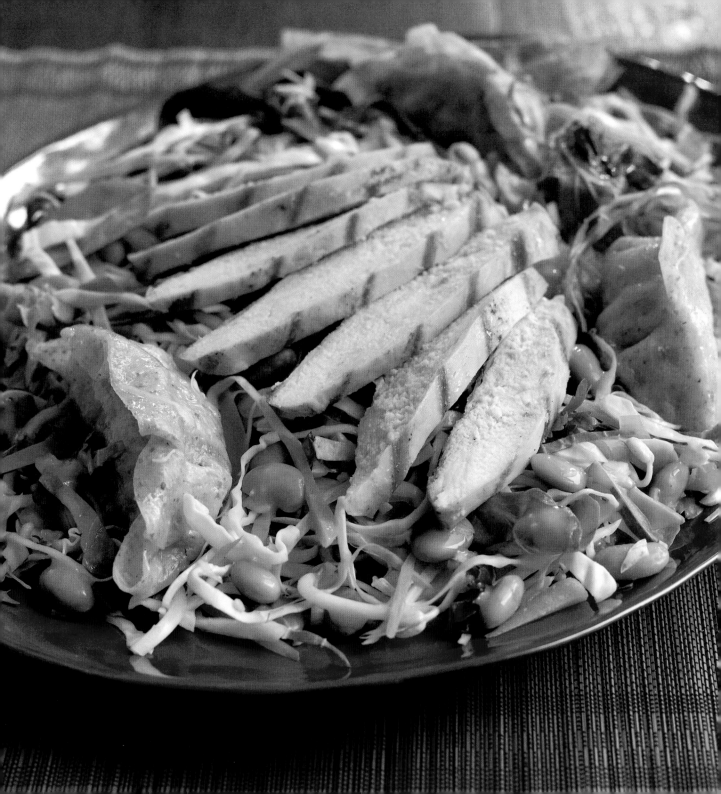

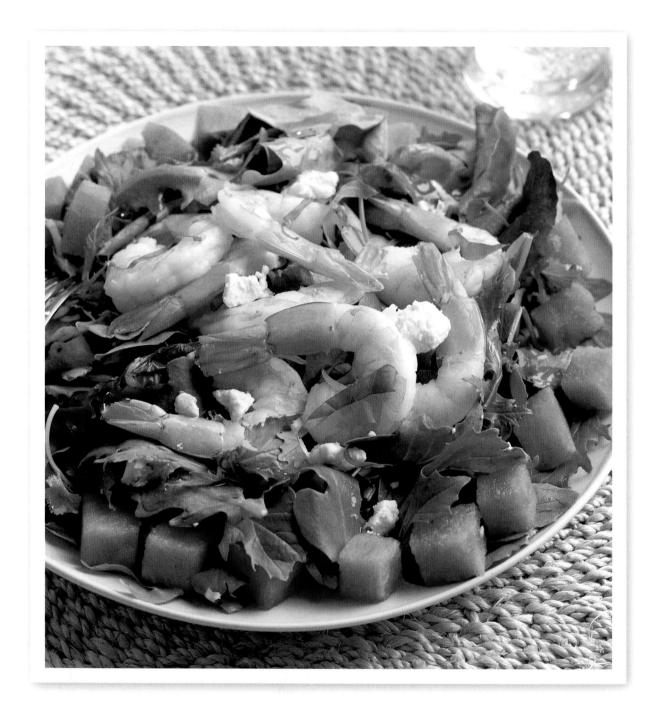

WATERMELON FETA SALAD

Last summer, I had to make dinner for a political candidate's campaign party where the guests had paid $5,000 per plate. Needless to say, I felt a bit of pressure to serve the perfect menu. When I went to the grocery store, I noticed that watermelon was ripe and in season, so I built this salad around it (though I served a homemade champagne vinaigrette instead of the bottled balsamic, which I've used here to keep things quick and easy). It was a huge hit, as the combo of flavors worked so well. Just be sure to get a really fresh watermelon. The cubes should be bright hot pink, almost red, not a dull pink.

4 cups loosely packed mixed green lettuce

6 medium basil leaves, slivered, or to taste

¾ ounce reduced-fat crumbled feta cheese

2 tablespoons all-natural, reduced-fat balsamic vinaigrette dressing (I used Follow Your Heart Organic Balsamic Vinaigrette Salad Dressing)

¼ pound large shrimp, peeled and deveined, steamed, and chilled

3 ounces (about ½ cup) ½" cubes watermelon

In a medium mixing bowl, toss the greens, basil, and about two-thirds of the feta with the dressing until well combined. Mound the salad on a plate. Top it with the shrimp and the remaining feta. Place the watermelon evenly around the edge of the plate. Serve immediately.

Makes 1 serving

Per serving: 275 calories, 31 g protein, 22 g carbohydrates (14 g sugar), 8 g fat, 3 g saturated fat, 179 mg cholesterol, 6 g fiber, 733 mg sodium

>>> TAKE IT TO GO! >>>

Pack the dressing in a small resealable plastic container, the watermelon in a small resealable bag, and the rest of the salad (shrimp included) in a resealable plastic container or a zip-top bag. Refrigerate until ready to enjoy, then assemble.

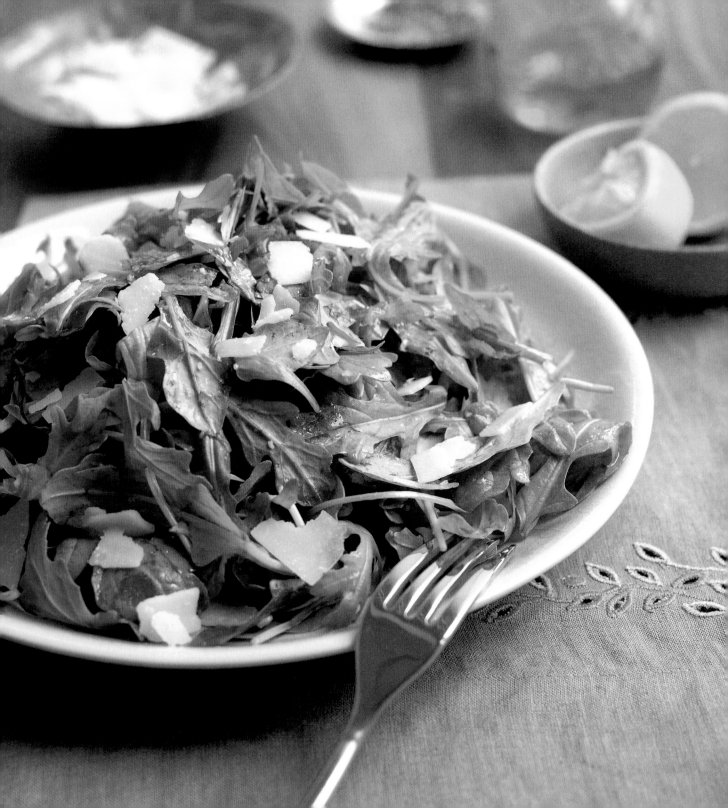

LEMON ARUGULA SALAD

Last holiday season, I gave out "homemade" gifts: bottles of Meyer lemon-infused extra-virgin olive oil with a little recipe card attached—for this recipe. I got rave reviews and thank-yous! Everyone loved that this salad was so flavorful and so simple to make.

It's really important to use fresh lemon juice in this yummy, large salad to create fresh, bright flavor. Pair it with half a sandwich, or toss in some lean protein like grilled chicken breast or shrimp to make this a full meal.

4 cups arugula leaves

1 tablespoon freshly squeezed lemon juice, or to taste

1 teaspoon Meyer lemon-infused extra-virgin olive oil

½ ounce Parmesan cheese shavings

A few sprinkles of sea salt (optional)

Place the arugula in a medium glass or plastic mixing bowl. Add the lemon juice and oil and most of the Parmesan, reserving a few pieces for garnish, and the sea salt, if desired. Toss to combine. Place on a serving plate and garnish with the reserved Parmesan. Serve immediately.

Makes 1 serving

Per serving: **114 calories, 7 g protein, 5 g carbohydrates (3 g sugar), 9 g fat, 3 g saturated fat, 10 mg cholesterol, 1 g fiber, 217 mg sodium**

MAKE A DIFFERENCE IN 20 MINUTES
Get in Line, Not Online

These days, online grocery store sites make it a breeze to order your weekly groceries with just one click. While the convenience of having nutritious foods delivered to your door is a big bonus, think about this: You can burn up to 52 calories in 20 minutes of grocery shopping. Considering that you probably spend at least 40 minutes at the store, that's a calorie deficit of 104 just by hoofing it around the aisles.

POMEGRANATE SPINACH SALAD

If you have trouble finding pomegranate arils (seeds), buy a whole pomegranate. You can remove the seeds yourself. You just want to make sure that you aren't wearing your favorite top when you do—pomegranate juice is as bad as red wine when it comes to stains.

In the Northern Hemisphere, pomegranate season is from September through February, but in the Southern Hemisphere, it's from March through May (they're often imported into the United States during those months). I've seen them at the grocery store in summer months, as well. But if you can't find the arils or a whole pomegranate, check for them in the freezer section. I prefer the fresh ones, but frozen will certainly work in a pinch.

---

4 cups baby spinach leaves

3 tablespoons pomegranate arils (seeds)

⅛ cup slivered red onion, or more to taste

2 tablespoons oil-free pomegranate vinaigrette dressing (I used Whole Food's Health Starts Here Low Sodium No Oil Pomegranate Vinaigrette Dressing)*

1 teaspoon extra-virgin olive oil

4 ounces sliced Essential Grilled Chicken (page xxii), or other low-sodium, lean grilled chicken breast

In a medium mixing bowl, toss the spinach, arils, and red onion with the vinaigrette and oil. Mound the mixture on a serving plate and top it with the chicken.

Makes 1 serving

Per serving: **287 calories, 29 g protein, 26 g carbohydrates (9 g sugar), 7 g fat, 1 g saturated fat, 65 mg cholesterol, 7 g fiber, 300 mg sodium**

*If your grocery store doesn't carry an oil-free pomegranate dressing, you can always use a light or low-fat dressing; just skip the 1 teaspoon of extra-virgin olive oil. Another option is to make a quick dressing with pomegranate vinegar and oil, or even swap in your favorite light balsamic dressing.

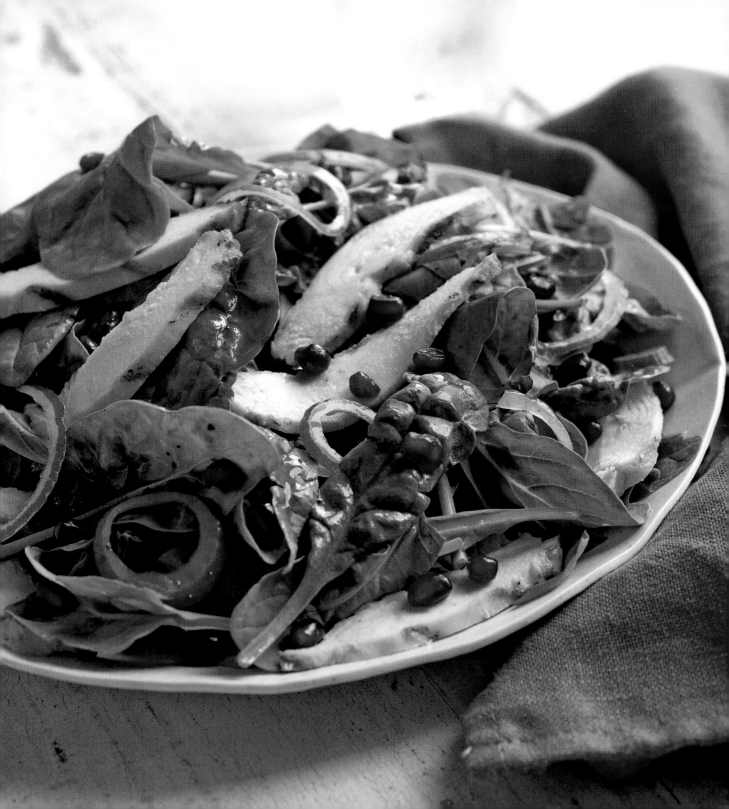

GAZPACHO QUINOA

This side dish is easy to throw together since all of the veggie chopping is done in a food processor. If you cook a batch of quinoa (see Basic Quinoa on page xxiii) on Sunday and keep it in your fridge, this salad will come together in no time at all on a weeknight.

4 medium cloves garlic, trimmed

2 whole scallions, trimmed and cut into thirds

2 medium tomatoes (about 8 ounces each), cored, quartered, and seeded

1½ cups broccoli florets

12 pitted kalamata olives

1½ cups cooked quinoa (page xxiii), chilled if necessary

1 tablespoon + 1 teaspoon freshly squeezed lemon juice

1 teaspoon extra-virgin olive oil

Sea salt, to taste

Fresh ground black pepper, to taste

To the bowl of a food processor fitted with a chopping blade, add the garlic and scallions and process until minced. Add the tomatoes, broccoli, and olives and pulse until the tomatoes are chopped and the broccoli is mostly the consistency of confetti.

Pour the mixture into a large glass or plastic mixing bowl. Add the quinoa, lemon juice, and oil and mix until well combined. Season with salt and pepper. Serve immediately.

Makes 4 (¾-cup) servings

Per serving: **140 calories, 5 g protein, 22 g carbohydrates (3 g sugar), 4 g fat, 1 g saturated fat, 0 mg cholesterol, 4 g fiber, 219 mg sodium**

Deni Hill SEASON 11

I'd never heard of quinoa until *The Biggest Loser*. But now I make it and add veggies to create a wrap sandwich with it, or have it as a side salad. I love it.

MUSHROOM ARTICHOKE COUSCOUS WITH LEMON AND PARMESAN

Make sure you use frozen artichokes for this recipe, not canned or jarred. Frozen artichokes have less sodium, and their texture works better in this dish. If you want to shave even more time off your meal prep, you can skip chopping the artichokes altogether.

Olive oil spray (propellant free)

1 package (8 ounces) sliced crimini or button mushrooms

1 cup (about 4 ounces) frozen and thawed artichoke hearts, drained of excess water

1 cup dry whole wheat couscous

1¼ cups boiling low-sodium vegetable or chicken broth (140 milligrams of sodium or less per 1 cup serving)

¼ teaspoon sea salt

2 tablespoons freshly squeezed lemon juice

1 tablespoon Meyer lemon-infused extra-virgin olive oil

2 tablespoons grated natural Parmesan cheese

2 tablespoons finely chopped flat-leaf parsley (optional)

Fresh ground black pepper, to taste

Place a medium saucepan over medium-high heat. When it's hot, lightly mist the pan with the olive oil spray and add the mushrooms. Cook, stirring frequently, for 5 to 7 minutes, or until lightly browned and the liquid that releases from them evaporates. Coarsely chop the artichoke hearts and stir them into the mushrooms.

Remove the pan from the heat and add the couscous and boiling broth. Immediately stir it well, until the ingredients are combined. Cover the pan and let the mixture stand for 6 to 8 minutes, or until the couscous has absorbed all of the liquid.

Fluff the couscous with a fork. Gently stir in the salt, lemon juice, and oil until well combined. Stir in the Parmesan, then the parsley and salt and pepper, if desired. Serve immediately.

Makes 4 (heaping 1-cup) servings

Per serving: 178 calories, 8 g protein, 28 g carbohydrates (1 g sugar), 5 g fat, 1 g saturated fat, 3 mg cholesterol, 6 g fiber, 318 mg sodium

>>> TAKE IT TO GO! >>>

This dish reheats perfectly in the microwave. Just store it in a resealable plastic container in the refrigerator or on ice until you are ready to enjoy it.

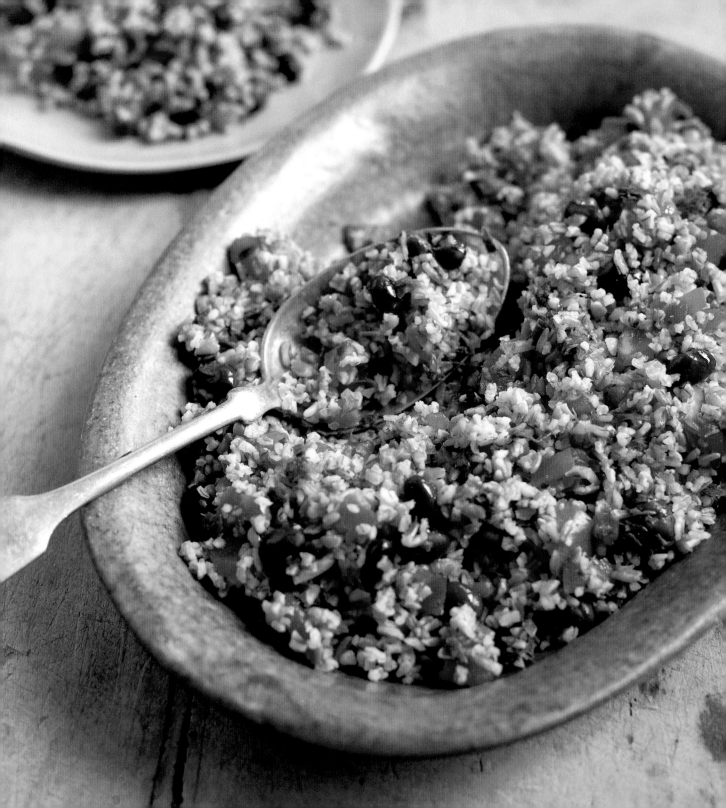

MEXICAN TABBOULI

When I write recipes, I often call for "fresh salsa," meaning the kind that you buy in the refrigerated section of the grocery store, not the jarred kind that you find in the center aisle near the chips. Fresh salsa has that fresh-from-the-garden taste, which really adds depth to dishes. It also tends to have a lot less preservatives than the jarred stuff. That said, always be sure to read the label.

1 cup dry bulgur wheat

1 cup cilantro leaves

2 medium cloves garlic

½ cup all-natural fresh salsa (the refrigerated kind, not the one in a jar)

½ cup drained natural no-salt-added canned black beans

¼ cup lime juice, preferably fresh squeezed

¼ teaspoon sea salt, or to taste

Cook the bulgur according to package directions, omitting any butter or oil. Spread the bulgur evenly over a sheet pan and refrigerate it for 10 minutes to cool, or until it is about room temperature.

Meanwhile, in the bowl of a food processor fitted with a chopping blade, pulse the cilantro and the garlic until the garlic cloves are finely chopped (but not so much that they're like paste). Transfer the mixture to a medium mixing bowl. Stir in the cooled bulgur, salsa, beans, and lime juice until well combined. Season with the salt.

Makes 4 (scant-cup) servings

Per serving: **157 calories, 6 g protein, 35 g carbohydrates (trace sugar), <1 g fat, trace saturated fat, 0 mg cholesterol, 8 g fiber, 172 mg sodium**

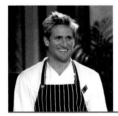

Biggest Loser Expert Tip: Chef Curtis Stone

If you're counting calories and you don't want to get into trouble with salads, try making your own dressings. A lot of people make the mistake of thinking they're eating a healthy salad, but the calories in a lot of dressings can really add up. So make your own! All you need is a little bit of vinegar and a little bit of olive oil.

LOSERS' LENTIL SALAD

This makes an excellent side dish at a picnic or barbecue and is a great to-go lunch. It's easy to prepare, especially if you buy presteamed lentils, which are available in the refrigerator section of many major grocery stores these days. Plus, it packs 10 grams of fiber, which means that it will fill you up!

2 cups steamed lentils, chilled

2 cups cubed red bell pepper

1 cup cubed English (or hothouse) cucumber

1 cup red onion, diced

3 tablespoons low-fat, low-sugar, low-sodium balsamic vinaigrette dressing (I used Follow Your Heart Organic Balsamic Vinaigrette Salad Dressing)

4 tablespoons balsamic vinegar

Sea salt, to taste

Fresh ground black pepper, to taste

2 ounces (½ cup) reduced-fat feta cheese crumbles

In a medium mixing bowl, toss the lentils, pepper, cucumber, and onion with the dressing and vinegar. Season with salt and pepper. Top with the cheese crumbles. Serve immediately or refrigerate for up to 3 days.

Makes 4 (1½-cup) servings

Per serving: 214 calories, 13 g protein, 33 g carbohydrates (10 g sugar), 4 g fat, 2 g saturated fat, 4 mg cholesterol, 10 g fiber, 279 mg sodium

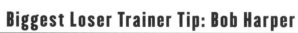

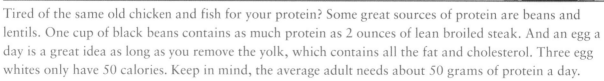

Biggest Loser Trainer Tip: Bob Harper

Tired of the same old chicken and fish for your protein? Some great sources of protein are beans and lentils. One cup of black beans contains as much protein as 2 ounces of lean broiled steak. And an egg a day is a great idea as long as you remove the yolk, which contains all the fat and cholesterol. Three egg whites only have 50 calories. Keep in mind, the average adult needs about 50 grams of protein a day.

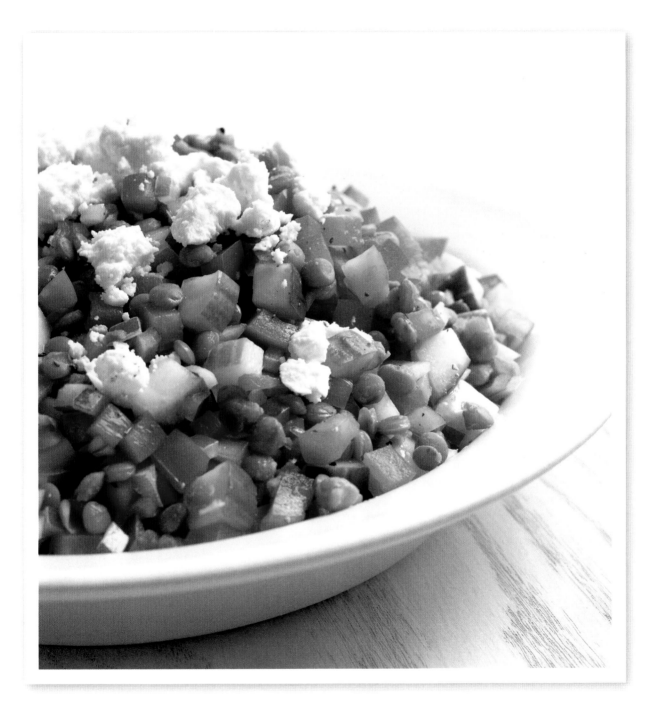

SUPER SIMPLE SLAW

I'm a big fan of hunting down natural low-fat sauces and spices that give healthy food a ton of flavor. Having lost 70 pounds, I've been committed to healthy decadent eating for a long time. And yogurt-based sauces like Greek tzatziki and Indian raita certainly help, especially when I'm in a pinch for a fast meal. They add flavor without adding a lot of fat and calories (though as always, be sure to read labels). Ethnic sauces and spices also inspire me to create new dishes and flavors. After all, who wants to eat the same old dinner every night?

1 cup broccoli slaw mix

1 tablespoon low-fat, all-natural raita (yogurt-based Indian sauce or dressing; preferably no more than 2 grams of fat per tablespoon)*

In a small glass or plastic mixing bowl, combine the slaw and the raita. Toss well to combine. Serve immediately or store in the refrigerator.

Makes 1 serving

Per serving: 33 calories, 2 g protein, 5 g carbohydrates (<1 g sugar), 1 g fat, < 1 g saturated fat, 3 mg cholesterol, 2 g fiber, 30 mg sodium

If your grocery store doesn't carry raita, check the salad dressings in the refrigerated section (usually found near the produce). Bolthouse Farms makes some really great natural, yogurt-based salad and cole-slaw dressings, as do other brands. Feel free to swap in one of your low-cal favorites.

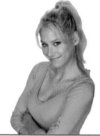

Biggest Loser Trainer Tip: Anna Kournikova

I'm a fruit and veggie freak. Growing up in Russia, I didn't see my first banana until I was 9 years old. It was green, and we put it on the windowsill and watched it ripen. Now I love to eat fruit whenever I can!

Biggest Loser Club Expert Tips: Greg Hottinger, RD

5 STEPS TO A HEALTHY SALAD

1. Pick Your Lettuce…

A great salad starts with great lettuce. Today you can find a variety of types of head lettuce, including green leaf, red leaf, and romaine. Once you've selected your favorite primary lettuce (or blend), you can greatly enhance the taste, satisfaction, and nutritional value of your salad by adding a variety of baby greens. Look for a simple blend of baby greens or baby spinach, or mixes that include fresh herbs like dill, parsley, and cilantro. As these delicious greens have grown in popularity, so too has the variety. Each new green that you add to your salad increases the variety of valuable nutrients to your diet.

2. Add Some Protein…

To turn a simple salad into a main meal, you'll need to add protein to meet your nutritional needs. Stay within *The Biggest Loser* meal recommendations by choosing a lean protein with 50 calories for every 7 grams of protein, such as salmon (50 calories per ounce), chicken and turkey breast (35 to 40 calories per ounce), tuna and shrimp (30 calories per ounce), and fat-free cottage cheese (30 calories per ounce).

Higher-calorie options include eggs (about 60 calories per egg) and lean red meat cuts like tenderloin (60 calories per ounce) and trimmed roast beef (45 calories per ounce). Instead of using cheese as a main source of protein (70 to 120 calories per ounce), use small amounts of feta, Parmesan, or goat cheese for flavoring.

3. Toss in a Little Carbohydrate…

You may find that a salad with a small amount of carbohydrate is more satisfying. Healthy carb additions include garbanzo beans, black beans, kidney beans, quinoa, wild rice, diced sweet potato, corn, peas, a toasted whole wheat pita, or a few whole wheat crackers on the side.

4. And Some Salad Dressing…

Remember that the wrong dressing can turn your salad from a healthy meal to a diet disaster. Every tablespoon of oil packs 120 calories, so use it sparingly. Dip your fork, choose a light dressing, or go with the calorie-free option of balsamic vinegar or fresh-squeezed lemon juice.

5. Finish It Off with Flavor Enhancers

When you add the right flavor enhancers to your salad, you won't need as much salad dressing, if any. On your next salad, experiment with fresh basil, cilantro, parsley, or dill. Add a few chopped artichoke hearts, sun-dried tomatoes, capers, roasted red pepper strips, or grilled pineapple. Or add some toasted nuts and seeds for texture and crunch, such as sesame seeds, pine nuts, pumpkin seeds, or chopped almonds, walnuts, or pecans (a tablespoon of each has about 40 calories).

"FRIED" MUSHROOM PARMESAN BAKE

This is a great vegetarian entrée or a fun side dish to accompany an Italian entrée. It's super quick and easy to throw together, too.

When cleaning mushrooms, don't run them under water. Instead, peel them or rub them with a damp paper towel to remove any dirt. Mushrooms are like sponges, so if you run them under water, they'll absorb a ton of moisture. The end result could be mushy or tough.

---

2 (8-ounce) packages button mushrooms, cleaned and stems removed*

½ cup all-natural marinara sauce (preferably low-fat, low-salt, no sugar added; I used Monte Bene Tomato Basil Pasta Sauce)

½ teaspoon dried oregano leaves

1 teaspoon garlic powder

1 ounce (about ¼ cup) finely shredded almond mozzarella cheese (I used Lisanatti)**

2 tablespoons all-natural whole wheat panko-style bread crumbs

2 teaspoons all-natural grated Parmesan cheese

Preheat the oven to 425°F.

Add the mushroom caps to an 8" × 8" glass or ceramic baking dish. Spoon the sauce evenly over the mushrooms. Sprinkle them evenly with the oregano followed by the garlic powder. Toss them gently to combine, flipping the mushrooms so they lay stem side down in the dish.

Bake for 15 to 20 minutes, or until the mushrooms are tender and mostly cooked through. Sprinkle the mozzarella, bread crumbs, and Parmesan evenly over the mushrooms. Bake for 4 to 6 minutes longer, or until the cheese is melted and the mushrooms are tender but not mushy. Let them rest for 5 minutes and serve.

Makes 4 servings

Per serving: 62 calories, 6 g protein, 8 g carbohydrates (3 g sugar), 1 g fat, < 1 g saturated fat, trace cholesterol, 2 g fiber, 110 mg sodium

You can save the mushroom stems to eat in a salad, or saute them and serve over a grilled buffalo steak or other extra-lean steak.

**If you can't find almond mozzarella, substitute the lightest, most natural mozzarella cheese you can find.*

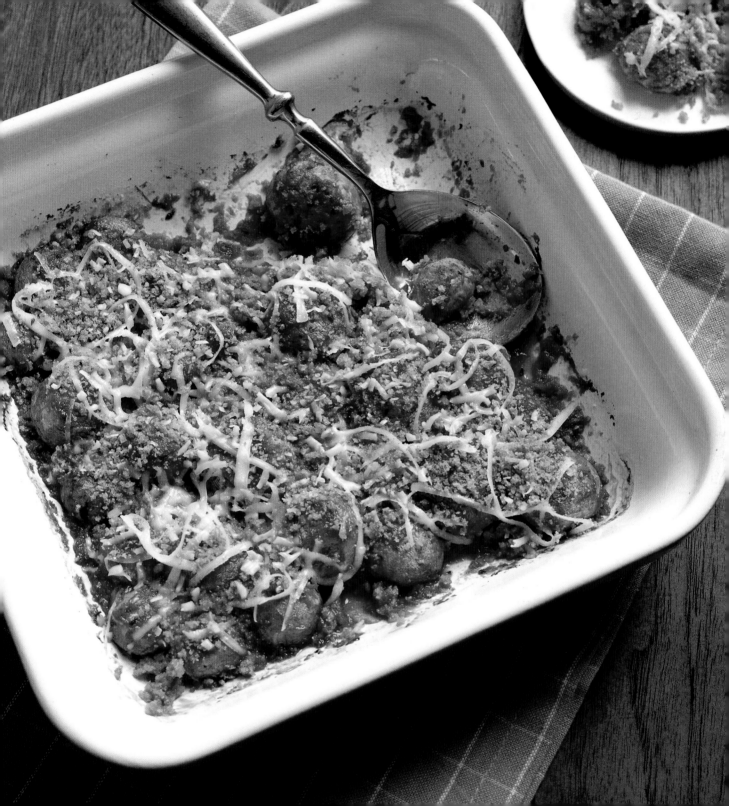

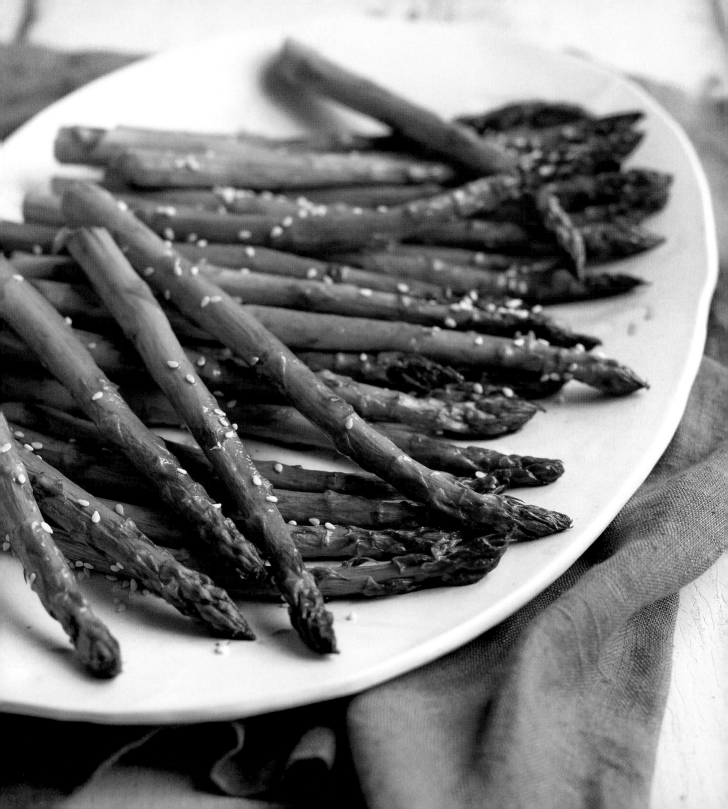

SESAME ROASTED ASPARAGUS

Just after I wrote The Biggest Loser Flavors of the World Cookbook, *I had a few of the contestants over for dinner to enjoy some of the Asian take-out favorites from the book. After planning the menu, I went to the grocery store. The asparagus looked amazing and happened to be on sale, so I threw together this dish at the last minute to serve with the other Asian dishes. It was such a hit that all of the contestants wanted the recipe—so I figured you would, too!*

2 **pounds asparagus, trimmed (about 1½ pounds after trimming)**

1 **tablespoon all-natural lower-sodium soy sauce**

2 **teaspoons roasted or toasted sesame oil**

2 **teaspoons sesame seeds**

Preheat the oven to 400°F. Line a large baking sheet with nonstick foil.

In a large glass or plastic bowl, toss the asparagus, soy sauce, and oil until the asparagus is lightly coated. Lay the spears side by side on the prepared baking sheet (it's okay if they do not fit in a single layer). Bake for 12 to 15 minutes, or until crisp-tender, rotating halfway through.

Transfer the spears to a serving platter and pour any liquid remaining in the pan over them. Sprinkle with sesame seeds and serve immediately.

Makes 4 servings

Per serving: **66 calories, 4 g protein, 7 g carbohydrates (3 g sugar), 3 g fat, trace saturated fat, 0 mg cholesterol, 4 g fiber, 121 mg sodium**

PARM-GARLIC ROASTED GREEN BEANS

Did you know that only one end of a green bean needs to be trimmed? Only one end has a stem, so there's no need to waste any of the smooth tapered end. Simply line up the stem ends and cut them off in seconds.

Though you can use a spatula or a couple of spoons to toss the beans, I like to use tongs. Not only are they efficient, but they tend to keep the seasonings on the beans—unlike other utensils, which can push them off.

---

1 pound green beans, trimmed

1 teaspoon extra-virgin olive oil

½ teaspoon garlic powder

1 tablespoon grated all-natural Parmesan cheese

Sea salt, to taste

Fresh ground black pepper, to taste

Preheat the oven to 425°F. Line a large baking sheet with nonstick foil.

Add the green beans to a large glass or plastic mixing bowl. Drizzle the oil over them, then sprinkle on the garlic powder and Parmesan. Toss until the beans are evenly coated. Season with salt and pepper. Toss again.

Spread the beans in an even layer on the prepared baking sheet so they are not touching (if possible). Bake for 6 minutes. Flip them and continue baking for 4 to 6 minutes, or until the beans are crisp-tender and lightly browned in spots. Serve immediately.

Makes 4 servings

Per serving: 46 calories, 2 g protein, 7 g carbohydrates (3 g sugar), 2 g fat, < 1 g saturated fat, 2 mg cholesterol, 4 g fiber, 32 mg sodium

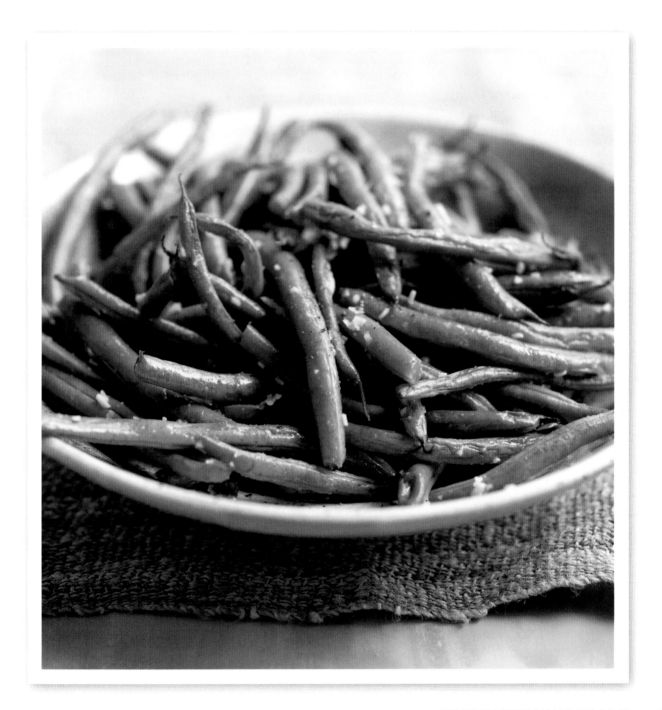

BROCCOLI WITH CARAWAY SEEDS

This is a great recipe for weeknights when you don't really want to do much more than steam broccoli. The caraway gives it a nice, unexpected kick. If you want even more flavor and have room in your calorie budget, toss the broccoli in a bit of light champagne vinaigrette or other mild salad dressing.

1   pound broccoli florets

1   teaspoon extra-virgin olive oil

1   teaspoon caraway seeds, or to taste

    Sea salt, to taste

    Fresh ground black pepper, to taste

Place a steamer rack in a large pot. Add enough water to the pot so that it reaches just beneath the rack. Place the pot over high heat and bring the water to a boil. Add the broccoli. Cover the pot with a lid and steam for 5 to 7 minutes, or until cooked and crisp-tender.

Drain the broccoli and add it to a large glass or plastic serving bowl. Gently toss the broccoli with the oil and seeds until well combined. Season with salt and pepper. Serve immediately.

Makes 4 (1½-cup) servings

Per serving: **44 calories, 3 g protein, 6 g carbohydrates (0 g sugar), 2 g fat, trace saturated fat, 0 mg cholesterol, 3 g fiber, 31 mg sodium**

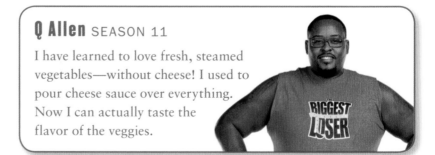

Q Allen SEASON 11

I have learned to love fresh, steamed vegetables—without cheese! I used to pour cheese sauce over everything. Now I can actually taste the flavor of the veggies.

Jesse Wornum SEASON 11

We were always rigging up stuff in the Ranch kitchen. One day, I cut up yellow and red peppers and some portobello mushrooms. I threw a little olive oil in the pan with garlic and onion, and then added the peppers and mushrooms. Then I threw in some scallops and seasonings, and added a dash of Worcestershire sauce. Delicious! That was my new dish.

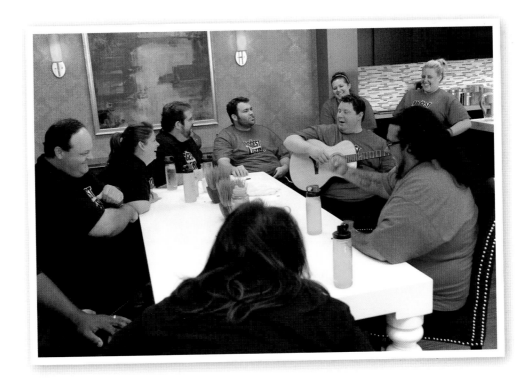

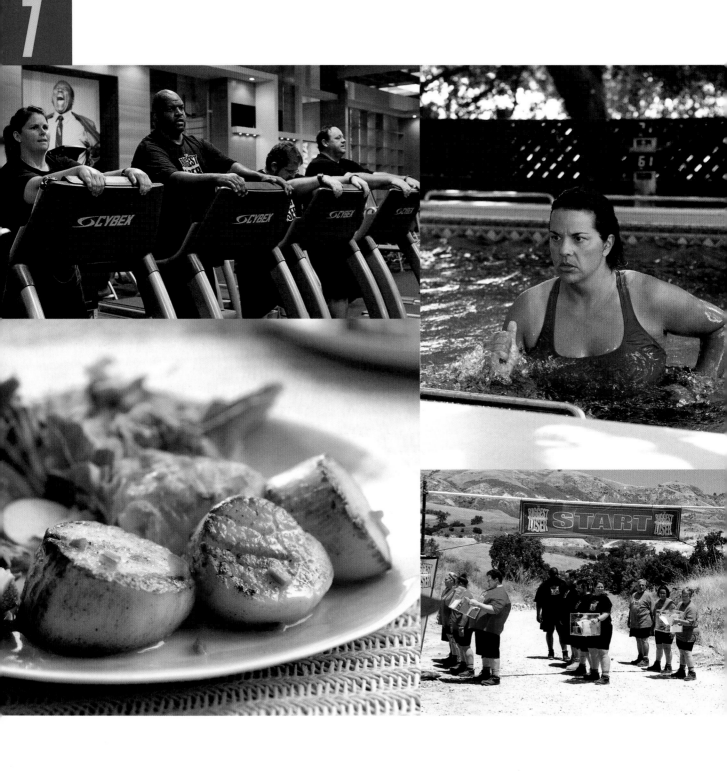

7

Mains in Minutes

The contestants on *The Biggest Loser* come from all walks of life, and over the years, we've seen some incredible demonstrations of talent, skill, and intellect. From teachers to lawyers to nurses to coaches to opera singers—the *Biggest Losers* are one talented bunch.

Except for one talent, that is. A skill that, season after season, most contestants admit to having little knowledge of (or are deathly afraid of): cooking. By now they know that when they arrive at the Ranch, there won't be any personal chefs greeting them at the door and asking for lunch requests. The contestants have access to a fully stocked pantry and a state-of-the-art kitchen 24 hours a day, but they are 100 percent responsible for cooking all of their own meals.

"I think it's really important for the contestants to learn how to cook on the Ranch because when they go home, they're gonna know what to do," says *Biggest Loser* Trainer Bob Harper. "They're not going to be able to go to some restaurant and say, 'I want to have the food that I had at the Ranch.' They're going to know how everything is prepared. Let me tell you, information is power!"

Many of the cooking-challenged admit that they've been relying on takeout, microwave meals, prepared foods, and restaurants to feed themselves and their families. And with jobs, childcare, errands, and a million other obligations to fulfill, they often feel like there just aren't enough hours in the day to prepare a healthy dinner at home.

They're not alone; many Americans feel the same way. In our time-starved culture, the idea of the family meal seems to have fallen by the wayside. But some research suggests that the more you make family dinners a priority, the more enjoyable—and healthy—your evenings will become. One study conducted by researchers at Columbia University found that the less often a family eats together, the worse the experience is likely to be—less conversation and less-healthy food. But the more often a family plans and eats dinner together, the more positive and healthy the experience is for everyone.

Other studies have suggested that kids who regularly eat dinner with their parents get better grades in school and are less likely to get into trouble. And spouses who eat together have a chance to reconnect at the end of a long, stressful day.

Season 12's Antone Davis says that when he feels his motivation to prepare healthy meals lagging, he reminds himself of what's at stake. "You have to remember why you are making the effort," he advises. "There are times you'll want to just sit down and rest and be idle, and you can do those things at the end of each day. But you're changing your life. You're making the effort each and every day to do that."

With Chef Devin's menu of hearty meals that you can throw together quickly like Easy-Breezy BBQ Pot Roast Dinner (page 163), Chicken Cordon Bleu Team (page 178), and 3-Ingredient Meatloaf (page 190), there are no more excuses for even the most time-starved among us to avoid the kitchen! In less time than it takes to watch a sitcom or wait for the delivery boy, you can create an opportunity to keep your family healthy.

Kelly Fields SEASON 5

One of my favorite quick and easy meals for two? Place 2 boneless skinless chicken breasts in a microwave bowl. Use a low-fat Italian dressing of your choice, garlic powder, and soy sauce. Pour the contents over the chicken and microwave for 6 to 7 minutes. Turn the chicken and repeat. You can dice the chicken at the 10-minute mark so it soaks up all the flavor. Serve with green veggies or on a salad.

COFFEE-CRUSTED CHOPPED STEAK

I've noticed a trend in restaurants of chefs adding coffee to just about everything—meatloaf, chili, steak, and many more desserts than in past years. Here's a simple, affordable ground beef recipe that will take mere minutes to throw together, yet is likely to be crave-worthy for die-hard coffee fans.

½ tablespoon finely ground coffee grounds (not instant)

¼ teaspoon sea salt, or to taste

1 pound 96% lean ground beef

Fresh ground black pepper, to taste

Olive oil spray (propellant free)

All-natural steak sauce (choose your favorite), optional

In a small bowl, mix the coffee and salt.

Divide the beef into 4 equal portions and shape each into an oval patty that measures 2½" wide and 5" long. Sprinkle the coffee mixture evenly over them, making sure they are dusted on all sides. Lightly press the coffee mixture into the patties, then season with pepper.

Place a large nonstick skillet over medium-high heat. When hot, lightly mist the skillet with the olive oil spray and add the patties in a single layer. Cook for 2 to 4 minutes per side, or until desired doneness is reached. Serve immediately with your favorite steak sauce.

Makes 4 servings

Per serving: 131 calories, 22 g protein, <1 g carbohydrates (0 g sugar), 5 g fat, 2 g saturated fat, 60 mg cholesterol, 0 g fiber, 208 mg sodium

MAKE A DIFFERENCE IN 20 MINUTES
Phone vs. Home

Ordering in dinner on a busy weeknight can seem like the fastest way to get a meal on the table. But think about it: Choosing a restaurant, placing your order, and waiting for the delivery person takes at least 20 minutes. The alternative? Take 20 minutes to create one of Chef Devin's healthy dinners for a fraction of the calories—and the cost.

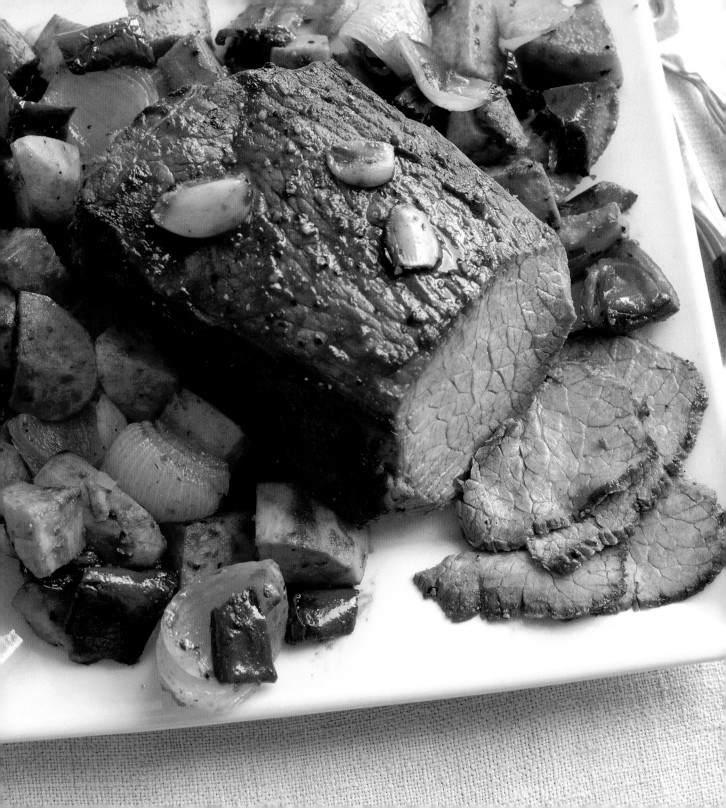

EASY-BREEZY BBQ POT ROAST DINNER

The most important rule when it comes to cooking lean cuts of meat is to not overcook them. Meats continue cooking when they emerge from the oven, especially large roasts. So, if you want this roast to be medium rare (130° to 135°F), remove it from the oven when a meat thermometer reads 125°F. Another important strategy is to tent the meat with aluminum foil after it's done cooking and allow it to rest for 10 minutes before you cut into it. By "tent," I mean place a piece of foil loosely over the roast (not sealed to the edges of the pan). When you slice it, slice it against the grain and make sure you slice it thinly.

- 2 pounds sweet potatoes cut into 1" cubes
- 2 pounds poblano peppers, stemmed, seeded, and cut into 1" cubes
- 4 teaspoons olive oil

- 1 tablespoon + 2 teaspoons salt-free mesquite seasoning (I used The Spice Hunter Salt Free Mesquite Seasoning Blend)
- ¼ teaspoon sea salt
- 2 pounds eye round roast, trimmed

- ¾ cup all-natural barbecue sauce, preferably sweetened with agave nectar or honey (I used OrganicVille Original BBQ Sauce)
- 3 small sweet white onions, trimmed, peeled, and quartered
- 8 cloves garlic

Preheat the oven to 450°F. Line the bottom and sides of a large roasting pan with nonstick foil.

In the prepared pan, toss the potatoes and peppers with 2 teaspoons of the olive oil and 1 tablespoon mesquite seasoning until they're evenly coated.

Rub the roast with the remaining 2 teaspoons olive oil, then the salt, and the 2 teaspoons seasoning. Place the roast in the center of the roasting pan, and arrange the potatoes and peppers around it, not under it. Drizzle the barbecue sauce evenly over the roast and vegetables, using a pastry brush to make sure the roast is completely covered.

(continued)

Separate the onions into layers. Scatter them over the top of the roast and veggies. Distribute the garlic cloves throughout the pan, placing 3 cloves directly on top of the meat. Bake for 20 minutes. Using a wooden spoon (so the foil doesn't rip), stir the veggies. Bake for 12 to 15 minutes longer, or until a meat thermometer reads 125°F when inserted in the center of the roast.

Take the pan out of the oven and transfer the roast to a cutting board. Tent it with foil for 10 minutes. Return the veggies to the oven if the potatoes are not fork-tender. Slice the meat into very thin slices against the grain at a 45-degree angle. Serve immediately with the veggies.

Makes 6 servings (4 ounces meat, 1½ cups veggies each)

Per serving: 474 calories, 39 g protein, 62 g carbohydrates (28 g sugar), 8 g fat, 2 g saturated fat, 62 mg cholesterol, 8 g fiber, 454 mg sodium

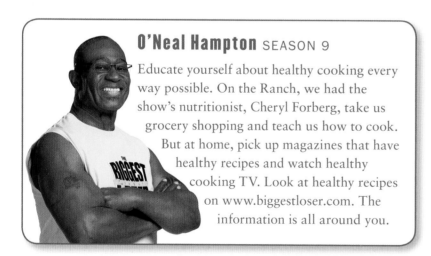

O'Neal Hampton SEASON 9

Educate yourself about healthy cooking every way possible. On the Ranch, we had the show's nutritionist, Cheryl Forberg, take us grocery shopping and teach us how to cook. But at home, pick up magazines that have healthy recipes and watch healthy cooking TV. Look at healthy recipes on www.biggestloser.com. The information is all around you.

BUFFALO BOK CHOY STIR-FRY

If you're not familiar with bok choy, it is a Chinese equivalent to cabbage and is found in most grocery stores. These days it's really quite common, and it makes an excellent addition to this stir-fry.

This recipe calls for roasted or toasted sesame oil. I strongly suggest that you use it (it should be brown in color, not clear or pale yellow) instead of regular sesame oil, as the roasted/toasted oil has a much richer and bolder flavor.

1½ teaspoons roasted or toasted sesame oil

1 medium (6 ounces) bok choy, end trimmed, cut once lengthwise and then crosswise into ½" pieces

½ small onion, cut into ½" squares (about ½ cup)

4 ounces buffalo sirloin steak, cut into bite-size strips

1 tablespoon all-natural Szechuan sauce, preferably honey- or agave-sweetened (I used San-J Szechuan Hot and Spicy Stir-Fry and Marinade)

Place a medium nonstick wok or skillet over medium-high heat. When hot, add 1 teaspoon of the oil, the bok choy, and onion. Cook, stirring occasionally, for 2 to 4 minutes, or until the veggies are crisp-tender. Transfer them to a medium shallow bowl. Cover the bowl and set aside.

Place the wok or skillet over high heat. Add the remaining ½ teaspoon oil and the steak in a single layer. Cook for 1 minute, flip the pieces, and cook for 30 seconds longer. Add the reserved veggies and cook, tossing with the meat, for 20 seconds.

Transfer the stir-fry to the bowl. Drizzle the sauce over top and toss to combine. Serve immediately.

Makes 1 serving

Per serving: 249 calories, 30 g protein, 11 g carbohydrates (5 g sugar), 9 fat, 2 g saturated fat, 47 mg cholesterol, 3 g fiber, 673 mg sodium

CHILI-RUBBED LONDON BROIL

I've now written eight cookbooks and think most of them (except The Biggest Loser Dessert Cookbook*!) contain a recipe for London broil. I just can't emphasize enough what a key dish this can be to beef eaters who want to be healthy and who are time-crunched. You can grill it in minutes, then use the leftovers in so many ways—cube it and toss into salads, slice it thinly for sandwiches, etc. At the end of the day, you'll have an amazing dinner followed by lean, clean deli roast beef that's virtually impossible to find packaged in a grocery store. Plus, you'll likely save a ton of money since deli roast beef is often quite pricey.*

1 teaspoon extra-virgin olive oil

1¼ pounds London broil, visible fat removed

2 teaspoons salt-free chili powder blend (I used The Spice Hunter Salt Free Chili Powder Blend)

¼ teaspoon + ⅛ teaspoon salt

Preheat a grill to high heat.

Rub the oil evenly over the London broil, then the chili powder and salt. Let stand for 5 minutes.

Grill for 4 to 6 minutes per side for medium rare, or until desired doneness is reached. Place on a large plate or platter and cover loosely with aluminum foil. Let stand for 10 minutes. Slice into thin slices against the grain and serve immediately. Or you can refrigerate and slice thinly on a meat slicer (or extremely thinly by hand) to use as deli meat.

Makes 4 (4-ounce) servings

Per serving: 125 calories, 24 g protein, 1 g carbohydrates (trace sugar), 5 g fat, 2 g saturated fat, 50 mg cholesterol, trace fiber, 273 mg sodium

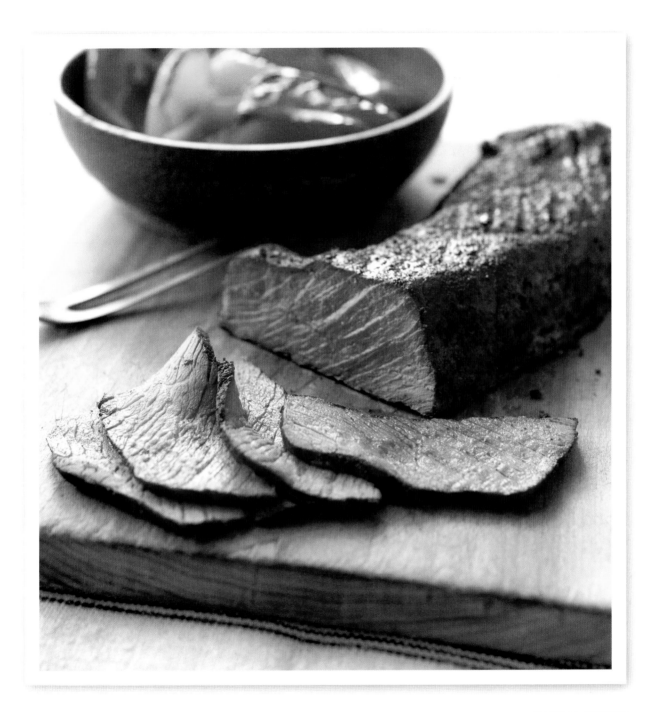

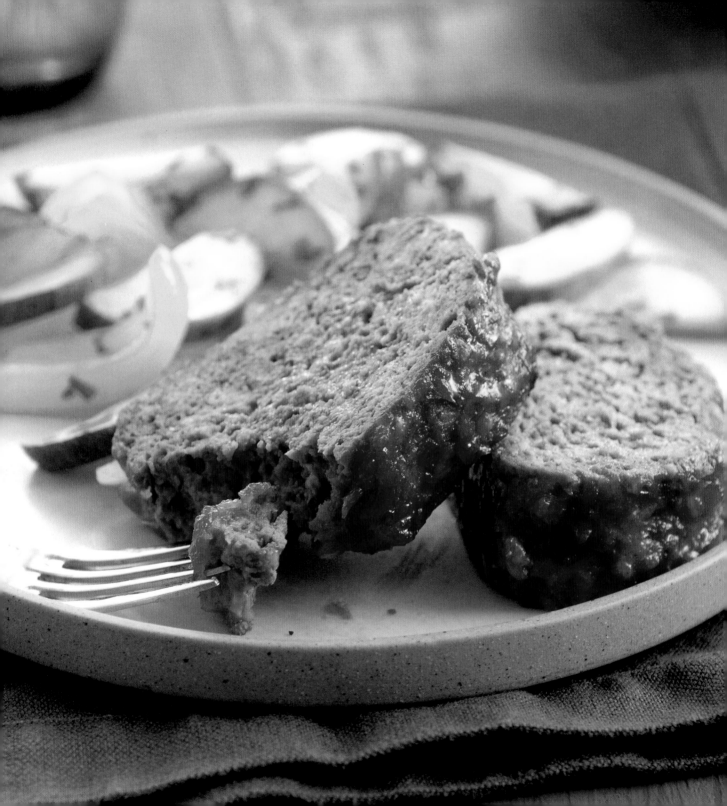

CHILI MEAT LOAF

This meat loaf is excellent reheated, and the Mexican flavors make it a great protein option for tacos, burritos, or other favorite south-of-the-border dishes. Your inclination may be to bake this in a loaf pan. While that is possible, I don't recommend it. The texture will be much better if you cook it as directed below.

Olive oil spray (propellant free)

1 pound 96% lean ground beef

2 tablespoons all-natural salt-free chili powder blend (I used The Spice Hunter Salt-Free Chili Powder Blend)

2 ounces (¾ cup) finely shredded, all-natural, low-fat Cheddar cheese (I used Cabot's 75% Reduced Fat Sharp Cheddar Cheese)

¼ teaspoon salt

3 tablespoons all-natural chili sauce, preferably agave-sweetened (I used OrganicVille Chili Sauce)*

Preheat the oven to 400°F. Mist an 8" × 8" round or square nonstick baking dish or cake pan with the olive oil spray.

In a medium mixing bowl, mix the beef, chili powder blend, cheese, and salt until well combined. Transfer the mixture to the prepared pan, shaping it into an 8" × 3" log that runs from one side of the pan to the other and is an even thickness throughout. Using a pastry brush for ease, spread the chili sauce evenly over the top and sides, making sure it does not run onto the pan.

Bake for 17 to 22 minutes, or until no longer pink inside. Let stand for 10 minutes. Transfer to a serving platter, cut into 8 slices, and serve immediately.

Makes 4 (2-slice) servings

Per serving: **172 calories, 27 g protein, 3 g carbohydrates (2 g sugar), 6 g fat, 2 g saturated fat, 65 mg cholesterol, trace fiber, 413 mg sodium**

The American-esque chili sauce used in this recipe is found near the ketchup, not in the international foods aisle where Asian chili sauce would likely be found.

PHILLY CHEESE STEAK PIZZA

I often use kitchen shears to cut tortilla pizzas. I find that it's easier to cut the topped tortillas into perfect slices with shears than with a pizza wheel or knife.

Note that it is important that you not use a tortilla that is artificially low in carbohydrates for this pizza. The low-carb ones contain additives and preservatives, and they will not crisp properly when cooked.

---

1 (10") all-natural sprouted grain tortilla or other (8") all-natural, low-fat whole grain tortilla (I used French Meadow Bakery Organic Sprouted Grain Tortillas)

4 ounces trimmed top round steak, preferably grass fed*

Olive oil spray (propellant free)

½ cup thinly sliced green bell pepper strips

¼ cup thinly sliced sweet onion strips

2 tablespoons all-natural cheese sauce or salsa con queso

Preheat the oven to 400°F.

Place the tortilla on a medium nonstick baking sheet. Bake for 2 to 4 minutes per side, or until crisp.

Shave the steak by holding a very sharp knife at a 45-degree angle and cutting slivers from the steak, basically tearing it until it's all shaved. It should be cut much more finely than if it were simply sliced.

Place a medium nonstick skillet over high heat. When the pan is hot, mist it with the olive oil spray and add the peppers and onions. Cook for 2 to 3 minutes, or until the veggies are slightly tender. Push the veggies to one side of the pan. Place the meat shavings in the pan and pull apart the shavings using 2 wooden spoons or spatulas. Cook for 30 seconds, just so that the meat is lightly browned on the outsides. Remove the meat and veggies to a bowl.

Spread the tortilla evenly with the cheese sauce, leaving a ½"-diameter border bare. Top that evenly with the beef, pepper, and onion mixture. Bake for 2 to 4 minutes, or until hot. Slice into wedges and serve immediately.

Makes 1 serving

Per serving: 335 calories, 34 g protein, 38 g carbohydrates (7 g sugar), 7 g fat, 2 g saturated fat, 50 mg cholesterol, 7 g fiber, 395 mg sodium

*Though you will only need 4 ounces of shavings, it will be easier to start with a larger piece of steak in order to achieve perfectly thin shavings.

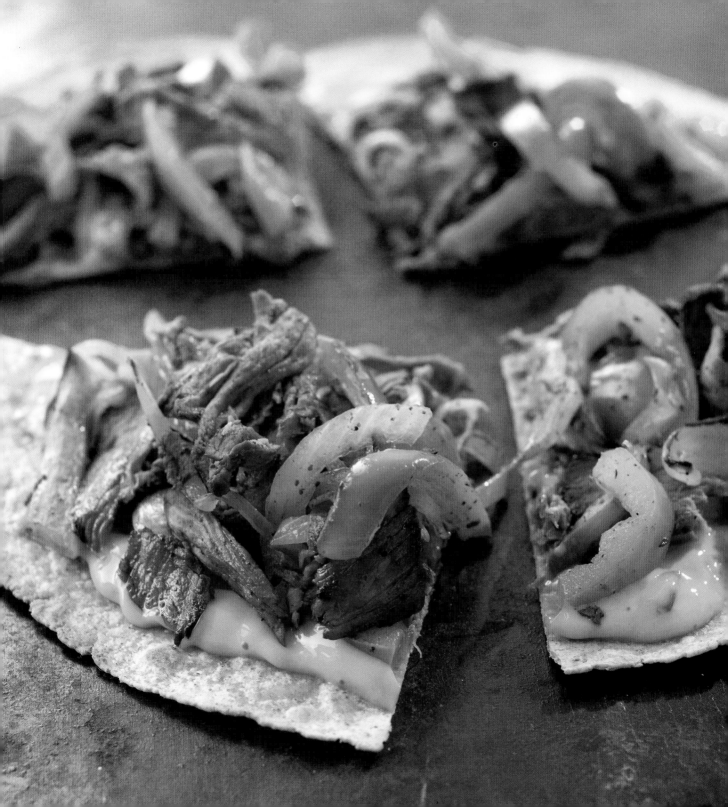

GRILLED BUFFALO STEAK WITH HORSERADISH CREAM

A 6-ounce buffalo sirloin steak has only 3 grams of fat, so I love to enjoy buffalo sirloin from time to time. But don't be fooled when going to restaurants. Just because you see the word buffalo on the menu doesn't mean it's always lean meat, especially in the case of buffalo burgers. Given that ground buffalo averages about 11 grams of fat and 190 calories for a 4-ounce serving, it's a safer bet to cook your own buffalo steak at home.

Though the horseradish sauce would traditionally be made with full-fat sour cream, I prefer good-quality Greek yogurt instead of low-fat sour cream. The texture of the yogurt is much richer.

½ teaspoon extra-virgin olive oil

2 (4-ounce) buffalo sirloin steaks

Sprinkle of sea salt, to taste

Sprinkle of fresh ground black pepper, to taste

Sprinkle of garlic powder, to taste

Sprinkle of onion powder, to taste

2 tablespoons fat-free Greek yogurt

½–1 tablespoon all-natural prepared horseradish, to taste

Preheat a grill to high heat.

Drizzle the oil over the steaks and rub to lightly coat them. Sprinkle with salt, pepper, garlic powder, and onion powder. Grill for 2 to 3 minutes per side for medium-rare, or until desired doneness is reached.

Meanwhile, mix the yogurt and horseradish in a small serving bowl.

Remove the steaks from the grill and tent them with foil. Let rest for 5 minutes. Serve immediately with about 1½ tablespoons of the horseradish sauce with each steak.

Makes 2 servings

Per serving: 149 calories, 26 g protein, 1 g carbohydrates (trace sugar), 4 g fat, 1 g saturated fat, 81 mg cholesterol, trace fiber, 76 mg sodium

Olivia Ward SEASON 11 WINNER

I love Italian food, and I'm not going to pretend that spaghetti squash is like penne ala vodka. But when you add marinara to it and a little bit of real Parmesan cheese, it gives you that luxurious taste, but you're still getting great nutrition.

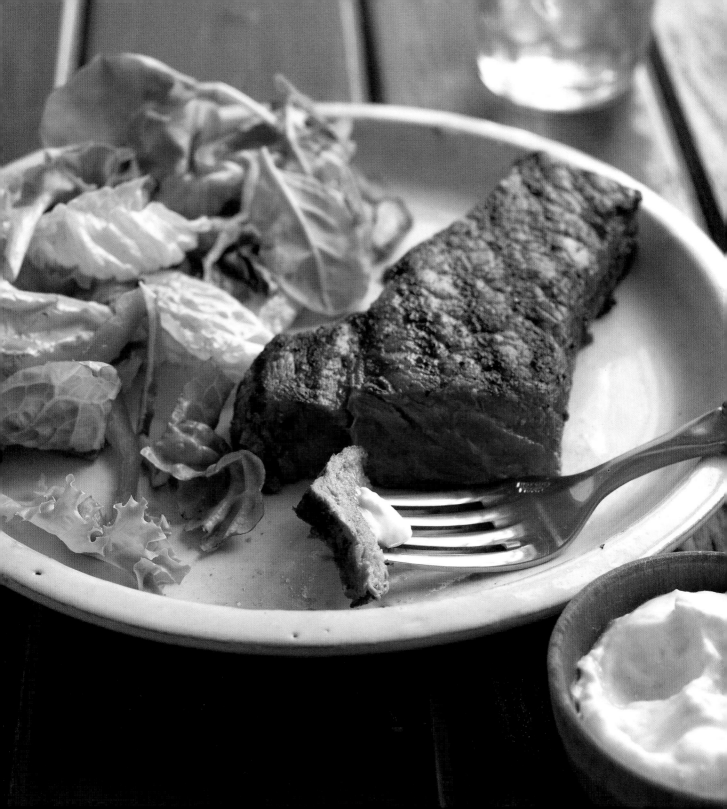

BLACK TEAM'S SLIMMER SUMMER SLAW WITH PORK MEDALLIONS

(Bob, Antone, Vinny, and Becky)

When I visited the Season 12 Biggest Losers for a cooking challenge, I have to admit I was impressed. The stakes were high: Each team had just 30 minutes to create a healthy, low-calorie, delicious entrée worthy of making it into this book. The winners not only got their recipe printed here, but also received a 1-pound advantage at weigh-in and a special lunch date with Season 11 winner Olivia Ward. In the end, the Black Team won with this tasty, satisfying pork dish that comes in at only 210 calories per serving. Congrats, Antone, Vinny, and Becky!

For the pork:

1 pound trimmed pork tenderloin

Olive oil spray (propellant free)

Garlic powder, to taste

Sea salt, to taste

Fresh ground black pepper, to taste

For the dressing:

¼ cup + 2 teaspoons red wine vinegar

2½ teaspoons toasted sesame oil

4 teaspoons nonfat Greek yogurt (the contestants used Fage)

½ teaspoon sea salt, or to taste

Fresh ground black pepper, to taste

For the slaw:

2 cups shredded green cabbage

2 cups shredded red cabbage

2 cups bite-size red bell pepper strips (about 2 small peppers)

1½ cups bite-size yellow bell pepper strips (about 1 medium pepper)

½ cup snap peas, thinly sliced on the diagonal

½ cup seeded, chopped cucumber

1 cup grape tomatoes (about 20 tomatoes), halved

For the sauce (optional):*

4 tablespoons natural, fruit-sweetened cranberry sauce (the Black Team used R.W. Knudsen Natural Cranberry Sauce)

½ teaspoon powdered ginger

Preheat a grill to high heat.

Lightly mist the tenderloin with the olive oil spray and season it with garlic powder, salt, and pepper.

Grill the tenderloin for 3 to 5 minutes on the 3 faces until it is just barely pink in the center (or a thermometer inserted in the center reads 160°F). Remove it to a cutting board or platter and tent it with foil. Let stand for 5 minutes. Then slice it into ½"-thick pieces.

In a small mixing bowl, whisk the vinegar, sesame oil, and yogurt until well combined. Whisk in the salt and season with pepper.

Meanwhile, in a large mixing bowl, toss the cabbages, peppers, peas, cucumber, and tomatoes with the dressing. Divide the slaw among 4 dinner plates, mounding it to one side of the plate.

If using, in a small microwave-safe bowl, mix the cranberry sauce and ginger. Microwave on medium power for 30 seconds, or until the sauce is slightly melted and warm.

Fan one-quarter of the pork slices next to the slaw on the empty portion of each plate. Spoon 1 tablespoon sauce on the side of each, if desired.

Makes 4 servings

Per serving (without sauce): 210 calories, 27 g protein, 13 g carbohydrates (7 g sugar), 6 g fat, 1 g saturated fat, 74 mg cholesterol, 4 g fiber, 368 mg sodium

Each serving of the sauce (about 1 scant tablespoon) has 28 calories and no fat.

Alfredo Dinten SEASON 10

I don't use any canned products or packaged foods at home. I'll use some frozen stuff because it's flash frozen, so it doesn't have preservatives. Cooking at home is the way to go. You know exactly what you're eating. You know the calorie count.

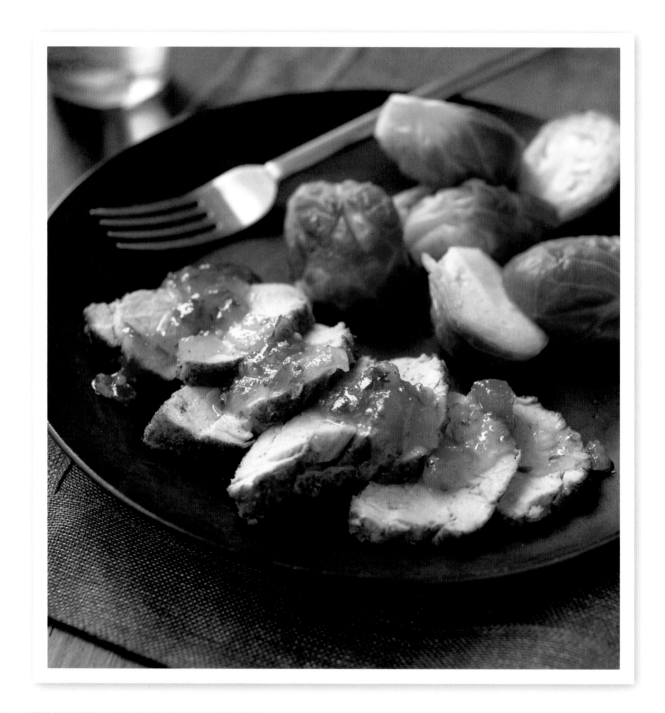

CURRY-RUBBED PORK TENDERLOIN WITH PEACH CHUTNEY

Pork tenderloin is another lean protein that is great to enjoy as an entrée—with the plan of using leftovers as super-yummy, ridiculously healthy sandwich meat for quick and easy lunches during the week. The Curry in a Hurry Pocket (page 120) is just one way to use this sliced meat. Feel free to make any healthy sandwich combo your heart desires!

1¼ **pounds pork tenderloin, visible fat removed**

1 **teaspoon extra-virgin olive oil**

¼ **teaspoon salt**

1 **tablespoon salt-free curry seasoning blend (I used The Spice Hunter Salt Free Curry Seasoning Blend)**

Olive oil spray (propellant free)

¼ **cup 100% fruit-juice sweetened peach chutney (I used Kozlowski Farms Peach Chutney)**

Preheat the oven to 350°F.

Place the tenderloin on a large plate. Rub it evenly with the oil, then the salt and the seasoning. Cover the plate loosely with plastic wrap and refrigerate for 15 minutes.

Heat a large ovenproof, nonstick skillet to medium-high heat. When the pan is hot, mist it with the olive oil spray. Cook the tenderloin for 1 minute per side, or until just browned on all sides.

Transfer the skillet to the oven and bake the tenderloin, uncovered, for 16 to 19 minutes, or until it is just barely pink inside or a meat thermometer reaches 165°F. Remove the pan from the oven and immediately place a sheet of foil loosely over the tenderloin (not over the whole pan). Let sit for 10 minutes (the internal temperature should be 170°F after it rests).

Meanwhile, spoon the chutney into a small microwave-safe bowl. Microwave on medium power for 30 seconds, or until hot. Set aside.

Transfer the tenderloin to a cutting board. Holding your knife at a 45-degree angle, slice it into thin slices. Serve immediately with 1 tablespoon of chutney per serving.

Makes 4 servings

Per serving: 184 calories, 26 g protein, 9 g carbohydrates (7 g sugar), 4 g fat, 1 g saturated fat, 81 mg cholesterol, <1 g fiber, 223 mg sodium

CHICKEN CORDON BLEU TEAM

Though this dish isn't exactly chicken cordon bleu—since the chicken isn't breaded and deep-fried—it's exactly as the Blue Team ordered it: healthy and delicious without breaking their calorie budget!

If your chicken breasts are thicker than ½ inch in any spot, it's best to pound them to an even ½-inch thickness. Simply place them on a cutting board, cover them with waxed paper or plastic wrap, and use the flat side of a meat mallet to pound them to the right thickness.

2 (4-ounce) boneless, skinless chicken breasts, visible fat removed, pounded to ½" thickness

Olive oil spray (propellant free)

Sea salt, to taste

Fresh ground black pepper, to taste

Garlic powder, to taste

2 ounces thinly sliced lean, nitrate-free ham

1 ounce thinly sliced all-natural reduced-fat Swiss cheese

½ teaspoon finely chopped fresh thyme leaves, or more to taste

Preheat the oven to 350°F.

Lightly mist the chicken with olive oil spray on both sides. Sprinkle evenly with salt, pepper, and garlic powder.

Place a medium ovenproof, nonstick skillet over high heat. When it's hot, lightly mist it with the spray and add the chicken. Cook for 1 to 2 minutes on each side, or until golden brown on the outside.

Remove the pan from the heat. Top each chicken breast with half of the ham and half of the cheese, making sure they do not hang over. Sprinkle each evenly with the thyme. Transfer the pan to the oven and bake for 4 to 6 minutes, or until the chicken is cooked through and no longer pink inside.

Makes 2 servings

Per serving: 193 calories, 36 g protein, 1 g carbohydrates (0 g sugar), 5 g fat, 2 g saturated fat, 90 mg cholesterol, trace fiber, 337 mg sodium

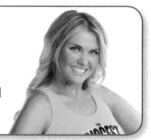

Sarah Nitta SEASON 11

It's so easy to make a veggie pizza on a whole wheat crust with lots of peppers, marinara, and low-fat mozzarella. I could eat that every day!

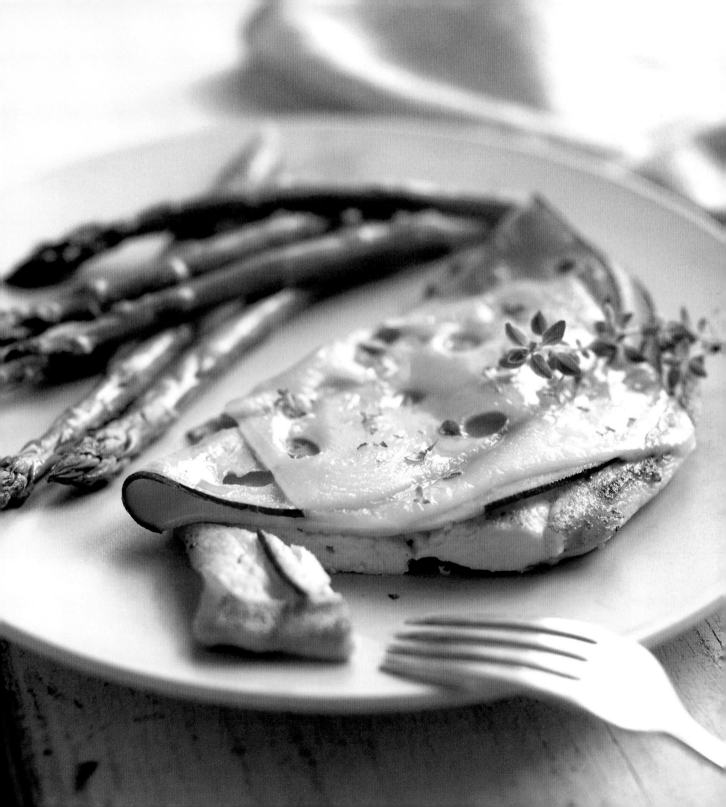

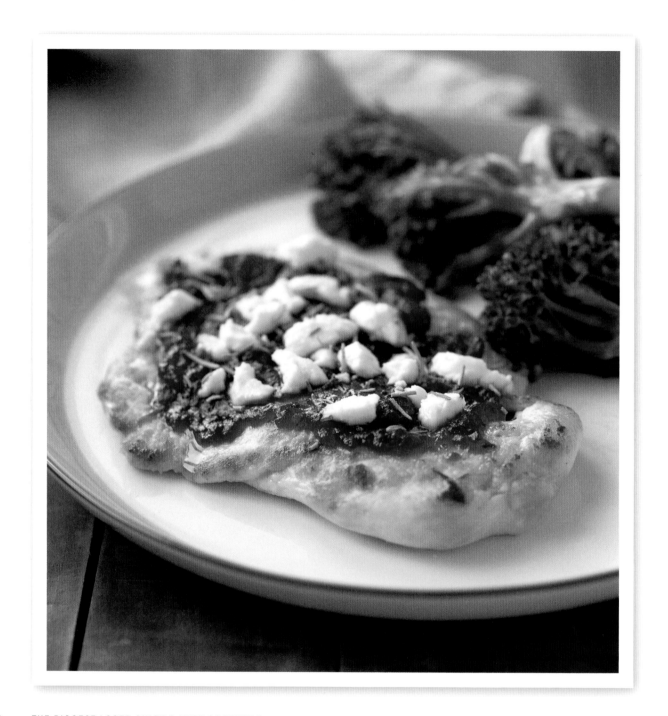

CRANBERRY GOAT CHEESE CHICKEN

This cooking method is by far one of my favorite for making perfect chicken. By searing in the juices and then finishing the cooking in the oven, you can't dry out the meat (just be sure not to leave it in the oven too long). Adding the cranberry and goat cheese will send it over the top, making it the perfect date-night meal or an impressive holiday entrée. Your guests will definitely think you spent way more time in the kitchen than you actually did!

4 (4-ounce) boneless, skinless chicken breasts, visible fat removed

Olive oil spray (propellant free)

Sea salt, to taste

Fresh ground black pepper, to taste

4 tablespoons 100% fruit-sweetened cranberry sauce (I used R.W. Knudsen Family Natural Cranberry Sauce)

2 ounces (about ½ cup) goat cheese crumbles

½ teaspoon dried rosemary leaves, or to taste

Preheat the oven to 350°F.

Pound each chicken breast to ½" thickness. Lightly mist both sides of each with the olive oil spray and sprinkle evenly with salt and pepper.

Place a large ovenproof, nonstick skillet over high heat. When it's hot, lightly mist the pan with the spray and add the chicken. Cook for 1 to 2 minutes on each side, or until golden brown on the outside. Remove the pan from the heat and top each chicken breast evenly with 1 tablespoon of the cranberry sauce, followed by one-quarter of the goat cheese (about ½ ounce each). Sprinkle the rosemary evenly over the tops.

Transfer the pan to the oven. Bake for 4 to 6 minutes, or until the chicken is no longer pink inside.

Makes 4 servings

Per serving: **192 calories, 29 g protein, 7 g carbohydrates (6 g sugar), 5 g fat, 2 g saturated fat, 72 mg cholesterol, trace fiber, 126 mg sodium**

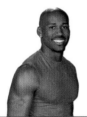

Biggest Loser Trainer Tip: Dolvett Quince

My favorite quick meal is some grilled chicken breast with quinoa and sliced tomatoes. Quinoa is full of protein, and it's delicious!

LUAU CHICKEN

It's best to pound your chicken to ½-inch thickness for this recipe. The chicken will cook faster, and you will be able to evenly spread your toppings on the chicken. To pound it, simply place it on a cutting board and cover it with plastic wrap. If you have a meat mallet, pound it with the flat side, starting with the thickest portion of the breast and working outward. If you don't have a meat mallet, you can use the back of a heavy skillet.

4   (4-ounce) boneless, skinless chicken breasts, visible fat removed, pounded to ½" thickness

Olive oil spray (propellant free)

Sea salt, to taste

Fresh ground black pepper, to taste

Garlic powder, to taste

¼   cup all-natural barbecue sauce preferably sweetened with agave or honey (I used OrganicVille Original BBQ Sauce)

4   slices all-natural canned pineapple slices in juice, drained

2   ounces (about ½ cup) goat cheese crumbles

Preheat the oven to 350°F.

Lightly mist the chicken breasts with olive oil spray on both sides. Sprinkle evenly with salt, pepper, and garlic powder.

Place a large ovenproof, nonstick skillet over high heat. When it's hot, lightly mist the pan with the spray and add the chicken, smooth side down. Cook for 2 to 3 minutes on each side, or until golden brown on the outside. Remove the pan from the heat and top each chicken breast with 1 tablespoon of the barbecue sauce, 1 slice of pineapple, and one-quarter of the goat cheese.

Transfer the pan to the oven. Bake for 4 to 7 minutes, or until cooked through and no longer pink.

Makes 4 servings

Per serving: 218 calories, 29 g protein, 15 g carbohydrates (13 g sugar), 4 g fat, 2 g saturated fat, 72 mg cholesterol, < 1 g fiber, 231 mg sodium

SASSY CHICKEN

Every once in a while, I spend an afternoon wandering the natural grocery store for products I've never tried. I read label after label, then take a pile of products home and experiment with new recipes. That's how I found the light cheese spread that I use here and in a few other recipes in the book. It's all natural and lighter than whipped cream cheese or the other cheese spreads in my grocery store. I was instantly hooked because it tastes great and a little goes a long way.

1 cup all-natural marinara sauce (preferably low-fat, low-salt, no sugar added; I used Monte Bene Tomato Basil Pasta Sauce)

4 (4-ounce) boneless, skinless chicken breasts, visible fat removed, pounded to ½" thickness

8 tablespoons all-natural light herbed cheese spread (I used Alouette Light Garlic and Herbs Soft Spreadable Cheese)

Preheat the oven to 350°F.

Pour the sauce evenly in the bottom of an 8" × 8" baking dish. Add the chicken breasts, flipping them to coat with sauce on all sides. Place them side by side, smooth sides up. Spoon 2 tablespoons of the cheese spread evenly on top of each. Cover the dish with foil.

Bake for 35 to 40 minutes, or until no longer pink inside. Serve immediately.

Makes 4 servings

Per serving: 194 calories, 29 g protein, 4 g carbohydrates (4 g sugar), 6 g fat, 3 g saturated fat, 81 mg cholesterol, <1 g fiber, 229 mg sodium

Allen Smith SEASON 8

My number-one diet tip: portion control! Cheese was my chocolate. I've cut back on the amount of cheese I eat and also made substitutions. Instead of always eating a full-fat cheese, I now try making recipes with low-fat versions.

KIDS' FAVORITE CHICKEN "PUCKS"

Remember when you were a kid and chicken patties were served in the school cafeteria? We used to call them "chicken pucks." Though that wasn't really a compliment, kids seem to love breaded chicken more than anything. Here's a much healthier, heartier version that moms and dads can feel great about serving and kids will love (as do the grown-up Biggest Loser *contestants!). Just be sure when you're buying the chicken that it's 99% lean ground chicken breast.*

Olive oil spray (propellant free)

1⅓ cups whole wheat panko bread crumbs

½ cup reduced-fat buttermilk

¼ teaspoon garlic powder

¼ teaspoon paprika

¼ teaspoon salt

¾ teaspoon fresh ground black pepper

¼ teaspoon cayenne

1 pound ground chicken breast

Preheat the oven to 450°F. Line a small baking sheet with nonstick foil. Lightly mist it with the olive oil spray. Place a sheet of waxed paper or parchment paper (about 12" long) on a clean, flat work surface.

Stir ⅔ cup of the bread crumbs and the buttermilk in a medium mixing bowl until combined. Let stand for 3 minutes, or until the bread crumbs begin to soften. Stir in the garlic powder, paprika, salt, pepper, and cayenne until well mixed. Add the chicken. With a fork or clean hands, mix the ingredients well. On the waxed paper, press the chicken mixture into 4 equal 4"-diameter patties.

Pour the remaining ⅔ cup bread crumbs onto a large plate. Carefully coat each chicken patty on all sides with the crumbs. Place the breaded patties on the prepared baking sheet. Bake for 12 to 15 minutes, turning halfway through, or until no longer pink inside. Quickly mist the patties with olive oil spray on both sides. Serve immediately.

Makes 4 servings

Per serving: **239 calories, 32 g protein, 21 g carbohydrates (2 g sugar), 3 g fat, < 1 g saturated fat, 68 mg cholesterol, 3 g fiber, 276 mg sodium**

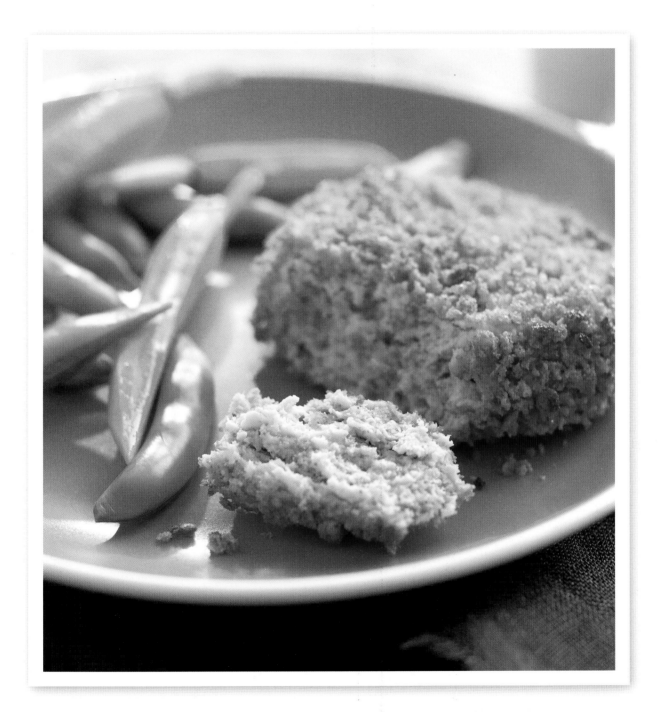

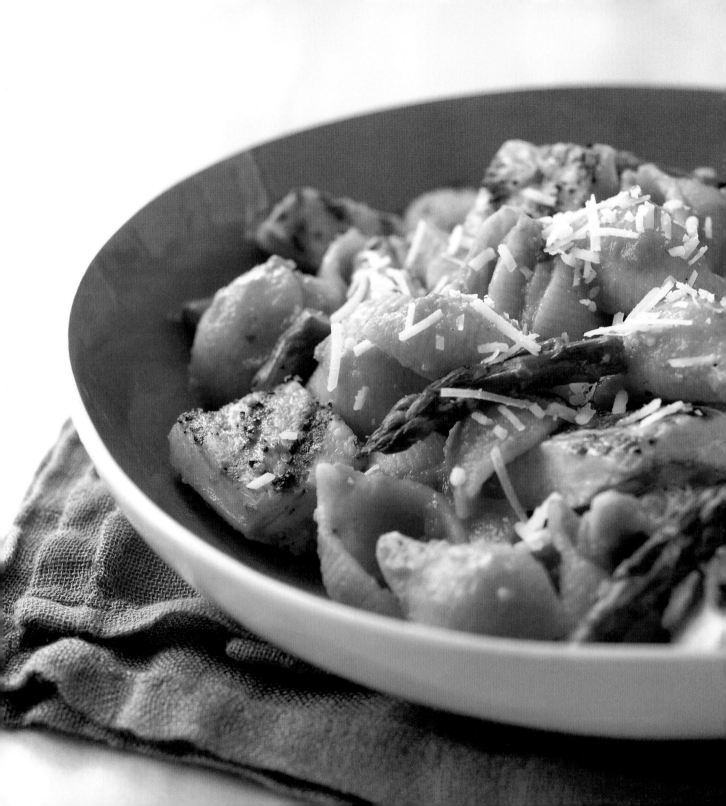

CHICKEN AND SHELLS IN VODKA SAUCE

The directions on many packages of pasta instruct you to cook the pasta at least a minute or two longer than I would ever cook it. So consider testing it for yourself. Set your timer for a few minutes less than instructed. Then strain out a piece of pasta or two, and run it under cold water to sample it. When it's arrived at the doneness level you most enjoy, strain it and add it to the recipe.

---

8 ounces dry whole wheat pasta shells

4 (4-ounce) boneless, skinless chicken breasts, visible fat removed

Olive oil spray (propellant free)

1⅛ teaspoons salt-free garlic seasoning (I used The Spice Hunter Salt Free Garlic Herb Bread Blend)

Sea salt to taste

Fresh ground black pepper, to taste

12 ounces trimmed medium asparagus spears*

⅛ teaspoon olive oil

2 cups all-natural low-fat vodka pasta sauce, heated (I used Monte Bene Low-Fat Vodka Pasta Sauce)

4 tablespoons shredded Parmesan cheese

Preheat a grill to high.

Cook the pasta according to package directions, omitting any oil.

Meanwhile, mist the chicken with olive oil spray. Sprinkle on 1 teaspoon of the seasoning, the salt, and pepper.

Toss the asparagus in ⅛ teaspoon olive oil and the remaining ⅛ teaspoon seasoning.

Grill the chicken for 4 to 6 minutes per side, or until no longer pink inside. At the same time, grill the asparagus for 3 to 6 minutes (depending on the thickness of the spears), rotating once until tender. Transfer the asparagus and chicken to a cutting board. Let stand for 3 minutes, then slice them into bite-size pieces.

In a large serving bowl, toss the pasta, sauce, chicken, and asparagus. Or divide them among 4 serving bowls. Top evenly with the Parmesan. Serve immediately.

Makes 4 (2-cup) servings

Per serving: **428 calories, 39 g protein, 52 g carbohydrates (5 g sugar), 8 g fat, 2 g saturated fat, 85 mg cholesterol, 9 g fiber, 309 mg sodium**

Be sure to buy at least a pound of asparagus. Per the instructions, you want 12 ounces to be the trimmed weight, not the weight before trimming.

INDIAN CHICKEN SIMMER

This recipe really couldn't be simpler. It's amazing how easy it is to yield perfectly tender chicken when it's "swimming" in sauce and baked in a covered casserole dish.

Though you may hit a snag finding the particular sauce I used in this recipe, don't despair. Feel free to use your favorite natural, low-fat, low-sodium sauce.

1⅓ cups all-natural low-fat, low-sodium Indian simmer sauce (I used Stonehouse 27 Cilantro and Coconut Sauce)*

4 (4-ounce) boneless, skinless chicken breasts, visible fat removed

Preheat the oven to 350°F.

Pour ⅓ cup of the sauce evenly in the bottom of an 8" × 8" baking dish. Place the chicken breasts side by side over the sauce. Pour the remaining sauce evenly over the chicken breasts, making sure they are completely covered (though they will not be submerged). Cover the dish with foil.

Bake for 30 to 35 minutes, or until no longer pink inside. Serve immediately.

Makes 4 servings

> **Per serving:** 205 calories, 27 g protein, 8 g carbohydrates (4 g sugar), 6 g fat, 2 g saturated fat, 66 mg cholesterol, 1 g fiber, 94 mg sodium

*Stonehouse 27 makes other delicious sauces in addition to this one. You can swap in any sauce you want, following the directions above, and you will get the same great results.

Antoine Dove SEASON 8

I've learned to substitute whole wheat pasta for white pasta in my favorite dishes, and sometimes I even substitute thin slices of zucchini for pasta noodles, to make a colorful and healthy pasta dish.

PRESTO PESTO TURKEY BREAST ROAST

This roast has become a go-to for many Biggest Loser *contestants. It's easy to make on a Sunday night, and then you can enjoy it for days cubed in salads, sliced on sandwiches, or tucked into lettuce wraps for a healthy snack or appetizer.*

Though it is possible to use a deboned turkey breast for this recipe, given that it is very lean, the turkey actually tastes better when prepared bone-in and then carved from the bone. Once it's cooled, I often rip the whole breast off the bone with my clean hands for easier slicing, though you can slice it right from the bone if preferred.

2-pound bone-in turkey breast half, skin and visible fat removed

1½ **tablespoons all-natural prepared pesto sauce (look for one with as little fat as possible, not more than 5 grams of fat per tablespoon)**

¼ **cup water**

Preheat the oven to 350°F.

Place the roast on a cutting board. With a fork, pierce the top (avoiding the bone) and the underside deeply about 25 times. Place the turkey, smooth side up, in an 8" × 8" glass or ceramic dish. Rub the pesto sauce over the breast meat (not over the bone), being sure to rub it on the underside as well as the top. Pour the water into the dish, taking care not to pour it over the turkey.

Roast for 45 to 50 minutes, or until a thermometer inserted in the thickest portion registers 175°F. Tent the roast loosely with foil and let stand for 10 minutes (the temperature should increase to 180°F). Place the turkey on a clean cutting board and carve it into thin slices against the grain to enjoy immediately. Or cut into thin slices or cubes to save for later meals. Refrigerate in an airtight plastic container for up to 3 days.

Makes 4 servings

Per serving: **172 calories, 34 g protein, <1 g carbohydrates (trace sugar), 4 g fat, trace saturated fat, 56 mg cholesterol, trace fiber, 129 mg sodium**

3-INGREDIENT MEAT LOAF

We've all heard that, in life, some things are greater than the sum of their parts. Here is an example: This meat loaf only uses three ingredients and can be put together in minutes, yet it yields a decadent dish that you would never guess is low in calories.

I wouldn't recommend making this in a loaf pan. The end result will be tastier if you use a baking dish or cake pan.

Olive oil spray (propellant free)

1 pound extra lean ground turkey

½ cup all-natural barbecue sauce, preferably sweetened with agave nectar or honey (I used OrganicVille Original BBQ Sauce)

2 ounces crumbled goat cheese

Preheat the oven to 400°F. Line an 8" × 8" square or round nonstick baking dish or cake pan with nonstick foil. Lightly mist the foil with the olive oil spray.

In a medium mixing bowl, mix the turkey, 5 tablespoons of the sauce, and the goat cheese until well combined. Transfer the mixture to the prepared pan, shaping it into an 8" × 3" log that stretches from one side of the pan to the other and is an even thickness. Using a pastry brush, spread the remaining sauce evenly over the top and sides, making sure it does not run onto the pan.

Bake for 23 to 27 minutes, or until no longer pink inside. Let stand for 10 minutes. Transfer to a serving platter, cut into 8 slices, and serve immediately.

Makes 4 (2-slice) servings

Per serving: 209 calories, 31 g protein, 13 g carbohydrates (11 g sugar), 5 g fat, 2 g saturated fat, 52 mg cholesterol, 0 g fiber, 317 mg sodium

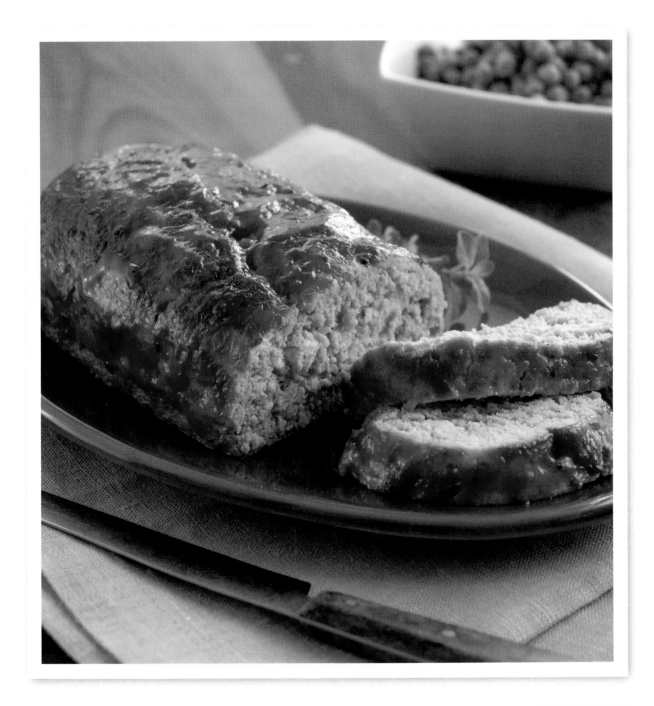

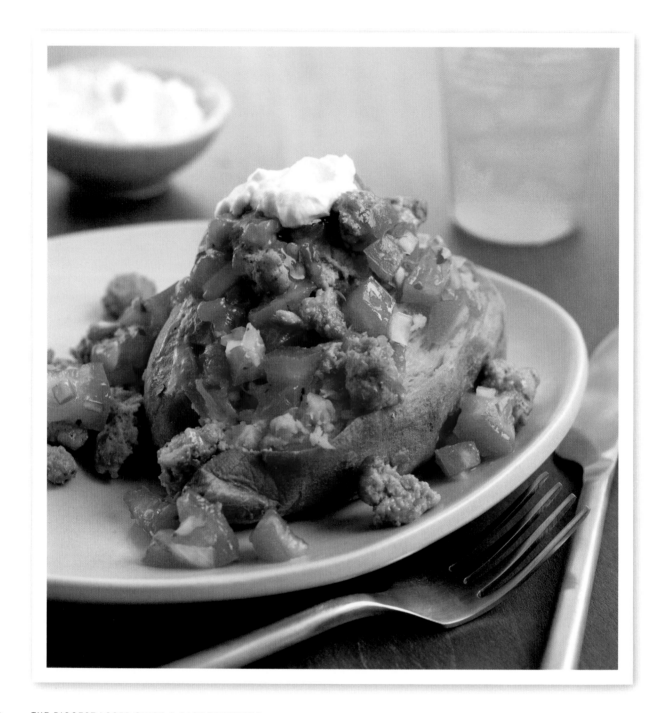

SOUTH-OF-THE-BORDER LOADED SWEET POTATO

When I'm cooking for myself, I prepare this potato with medium salsa, and it has a nice kick. Feel free to use mild or hot, as many of the contestants do.

When it comes to topping the potato with salsa, start out with ⅓ cup of fresh salsa and drain the liquid from it. It will likely only be about ¼ cup (maybe a bit more) in the end. Note that the toppings won't fit inside the potato—they will spill out over the top, making it even more decadent to eat!

---

1 (8-ounce) sweet potato

4 ounces extra-lean ground turkey

¾ teaspoon all-natural salt-free fajita or Southwest seasoning

Olive oil spray (propellant free)

⅓ cup fresh salsa, drained

2 tablespoons jarred all-natural roasted green salsa

2 tablespoons fat-free Greek yogurt

Using a fork, poke the potato 5 times on all sides and place it in a microwave-safe bowl or dish. Cover the dish loosely with a paper towel. Microwave it on high for 3 minutes. Carefully flip the potato (it will be very hot) and continue microwaving for 2 to 4 minutes longer, or until cooked and tender.

Meanwhile, in a small bowl, mix the turkey and seasoning.

Place a small nonstick skillet over medium-high heat. When hot, lightly mist it with the olive oil spray. Cook the turkey for 3 to 4 minutes, or until no longer pink, breaking it into bite-size chunks as you do.

Cut an opening in the potato that stretches 1" from each end of the potato and deep enough to open the potato completely without cutting it in half. Put it in a medium shallow bowl. Stuff the potato with the fresh salsa, then the turkey, then the green salsa. Top it with the yogurt. Serve immediately.

Makes 1 serving

Per serving: 342 calories, 35 g protein, 47 g carbohydrates (13 g sugar), 2 g fat, trace saturated fat, 45 mg cholesterol, 8 g fiber, 304 mg sodium

CRUSTLESS TURKEY "PIZZA"

This dish is the furthest thing from a gourmet meal, yet it is extremely satisfying for low-carbers and the gluten-intolerant, and it's always a hit with kids (though you may want to omit the red-pepper flakes for them). Have your kids help you assemble it to get the job done even quicker, and teach them about healthy eating.

Olive oil spray (propellant free)

1 pound ground extra lean turkey breast

¾ cup all-natural marinara sauce (preferably low-fat, low-salt, no sugar added; I used Monte Bene Tomato Basil Pasta Sauce)

½ teaspoon dried oregano

⅛ teaspoon red-pepper flakes, or more to taste

3 ounces (¾ cup) finely shredded almond mozzarella cheese (I use Lisanatti)*

Preheat the oven to 400°F. Mist an 11" × 7" baking dish with the olive oil spray.

Spread the turkey evenly in the baking dish. Spoon the sauce into the center. Then using the back of a spoon, spread the sauce evenly over all but the outer ½", like you're adding sauce to a pizza crust. Sprinkle the oregano, pepper flakes, and then the cheese evenly over the sauce.

Bake for 13 to 15 minutes, or until the turkey is no longer pink in the center. If there is liquid surrounding it, carefully pour as much of it out of the dish as you can without the sauce and cheese sliding. Slice it into 8 even rectangles and serve immediately.

Makes 4 (2-slice) servings

Per serving: 174 calories, 34 g protein, 4 g carbohydrates (1 g sugar), 3 g fat, trace saturated fat, 45 mg cholesterol, 1 g fiber, 279 mg sodium

If you can find preshredded cheese, buy that to save time. If not, be sure to shred the cheese finely. By shredding it finely, not only will it melt better, you will need less.

MOLASSES MUSTARD SALMON

When shopping for salmon, there are a couple of things to remember. First, be sure to ask your fishmonger for the wide part of the fish's body—it tastes better. Second, always try to purchase wild-caught salmon. It's better for you than the farmed variety, and it tastes better, too. Finally, if you're buying packaged fresh or frozen fish, be sure the tail isn't tucked underneath the body of the fish, making it look thick. Thicker pieces are more premium, so sometimes grocery stores need to help along the sales of the tail pieces.

Olive oil spray (propellant free)

3 tablespoons all-natural Dijon mustard (make sure it does not have sugar in it; I used Westbrae Natural Dijon Style Mustard)

1 tablespoon molasses

4 (4-ounce) salmon fillets, preferably wild-caught

Sea salt, to taste

Fresh ground black pepper, to taste

Preheat the oven to 400°F. Mist an 8" × 8" baking dish or pan with the olive oil spray.*

In a small bowl, whisk the mustard and molasses together until well-combined.

Place the salmon fillets in the prepared baking dish. Using a pastry brush for ease, brush the molasses mixture evenly over the tops and sides of all 4 fillets. Sprinkle with salt and pepper. Cook for 10 to 12 minutes, or until the fish flakes easily with a fork.

Makes 4 servings

Per serving: 223 calories, 23 g protein, 5 g carbohydrates (3 g sugar), 12 g fat, 2 g saturated fat, 67 mg cholesterol, 193 mg sodium, 0 g fiber

*Be sure to use a pan or dish with an edge so that the juice from the salmon does not drip into your oven.

TAKE IT TO GO!

Although some people might find it odd to eat this salmon cold, I really enjoy it. It makes a great lunch or, in a smaller portion, pre-gym snack. If you want to take it on the go, just pack it in a resealable plastic container and store it in the refrigerator or on ice until it's time to enjoy.

FRESH-AS-CAN-BE JALAPEÑO LIME SCALLOPS

These scallops provide a fresh burst of flavor. The key is to make sure you get good caramelization (a nice, even browning) on each side. To do that, be sure that the scallops are free of excess moisture and the pan is nice and hot.

Note that if you do not want to invest in the jalapeño lime olive oil, it is possible to simply use a good extra-virgin olive oil in its place. If you opt to do that, you might want to increase the fresh lime and jalapeño a bit.

1 pound sea scallops

Sea salt, to taste

2 teaspoons jalapeño lime-infused extra-virgin olive oil, divided

2 tablespoons freshly squeezed lime juice, or more to taste

1 teaspoon finely chopped fresh jalapeño chile pepper

Pat the scallops dry with a paper towel to remove any excess moisture. In a small mixing bowl, toss the scallops with 1 teaspoon of olive oil until evenly coated. Season with salt and toss again.

Place a large nonstick skillet over high heat. When hot, working in batches if necessary, add the scallops in a single layer, not touching. Cook for 2 to 3 minutes per side, or until golden brown on the outsides and barely translucent inside.

Meanwhile, in a small bowl, stir together the remaining teaspoon of olive oil and lime juice.

Divide the scallops among 4 serving plates. Pour the sauce evenly over them, then sprinkle on the pepper. Serve immediately.

Makes 4 servings

Per serving: **122 calories, 19 g protein, 3 g carbohydrates (trace sugar), 3 g fat, trace saturated fat, 37 mg cholesterol, trace fiber, 183 mg sodium**

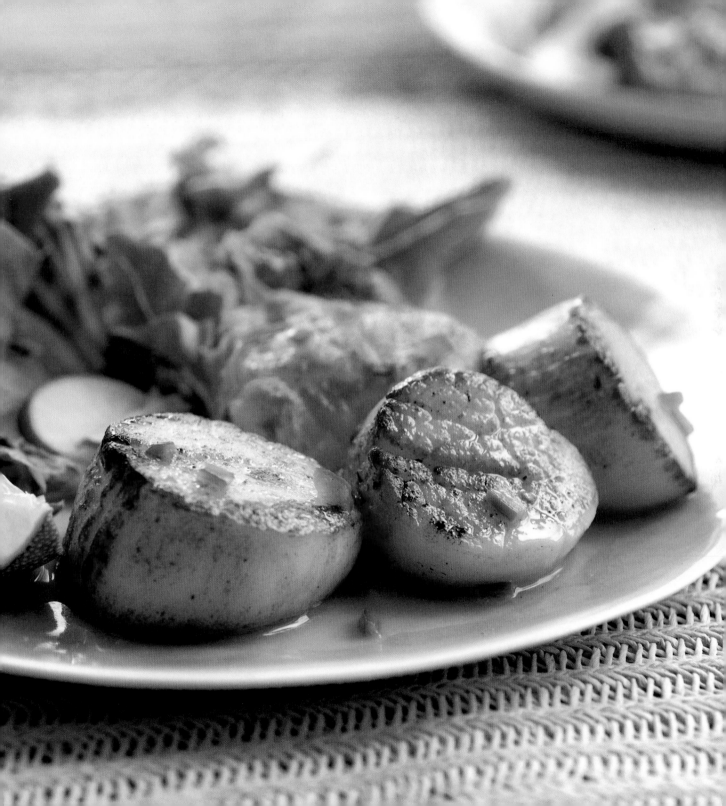

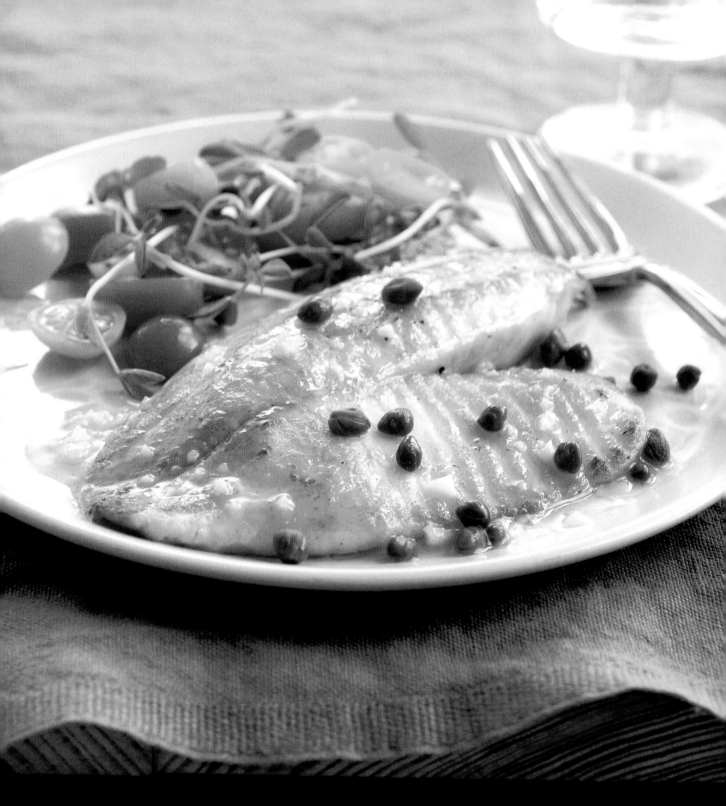

TIME-CRUNCHED TILAPIA PICCATA

Tilapia fillets vary in size, so you might need 1½ or even 2 fillets for this recipe. Just watch them closely in the last couple of minutes of cooking if they're not uniform in size, so you can remove the smaller fillet as soon as it's done. Note that this recipe is really easy to double or quadruple if you're cooking for a crowd. Just make sure to use a pan that's large enough to accommodate the fillets in a single layer. If the fillets overlap, they're not likely to ever get a nice golden brown exterior.

4 ounces tilapia fillet(s)

Sea salt, to taste

Fresh ground black pepper, to taste

1 teaspoon all-natural whipped buttery spread (I used Earth Balance Whipped Organic Buttery Spread)

1 teaspoon minced garlic

Olive oil spray (propellant free)

1 tablespoon freshly squeezed lemon juice

1 tablespoon drained capers

Season the fillet(s) with salt and pepper.

To a small microwave-safe bowl, add the buttery spread and garlic.

Place a small nonstick skillet over medium-high heat. When it's hot, lightly mist it with the olive oil spray, then add the fillet(s) side by side. Cook for 2 to 3 minutes per side, or until golden brown on the outside and the fish flakes.

Meanwhile, microwave the butter mixture on high for 20 to 30 seconds, or until the buttery spread is melted. Stir in the lemon juice.

Transfer the fillet(s) to a serving plate. Pour the lemon butter mixture over top, then sprinkle on the capers. Serve immediately.

Makes 1 serving

Per serving: **148 calories, 23 g protein, 3 g carbohydrates (trace sugar), 5 g fat, 2 g saturated fat, 57 mg cholesterol, trace fiber, 348 mg sodium**

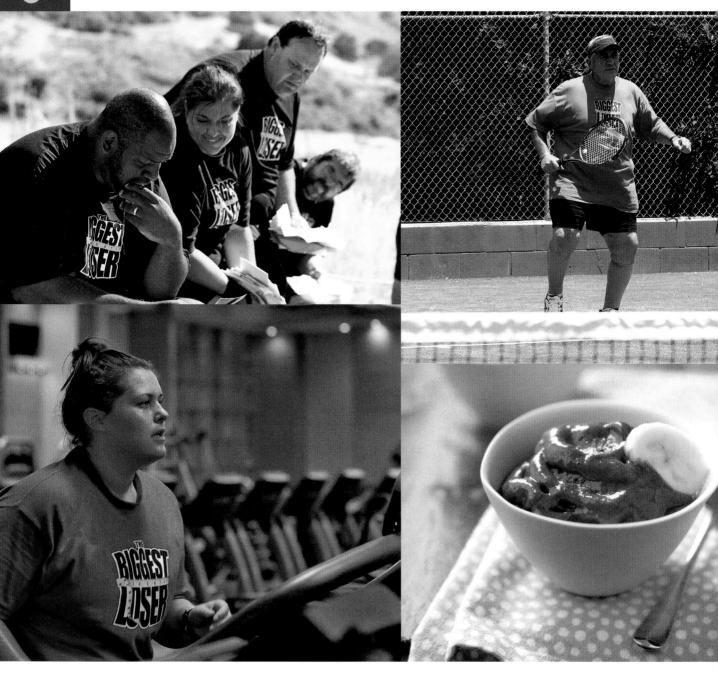

8

Lickety-Split
Sweet Bites and Sips

When it comes to healthy treats and weight loss, there are three common misconceptions. The first is that creating your own healthy desserts is too hard—it requires a lot of time in the kitchen and a lot of hard-to-find ingredients. The second is that sin-free sweets just don't taste as good as the real thing. And the third? That if you're trying to lose weight, you probably shouldn't be indulging your sweet tooth to begin with.

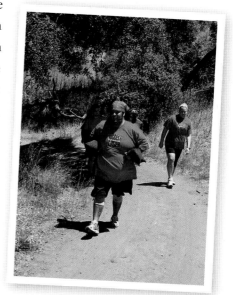

Well, with Chef Devin's quick and easy desserts, you don't have to worry about spending a lot of time in the kitchen or having to find rare ingredients. Most of the desserts in the pages that follow are made from ingredients you can find at your local grocery store or health food store, and they can be thrown together in a snap (no hourlong oven time required).

And while it's true that sweets should be limited when you're trying to lose weight, it's important to allow yourself a sweet nothing every now and then, so that you don't feel deprived.

"For me, the key to maintaining a substantial weight loss for 17 years has been regularly allowing myself healthy indulgences," says Chef Devin. "People who are trying to lose weight often think that they can never eat sweets again. But you can satisfy your sweet cravings in a multitude of ways without breaking your calorie budget."

Biggest Loser trainer Anna Kournikova agrees. Like Chef Devin, she loves her chocolate. "My philosophy is that you can indulge, but in moderation. Have a small piece of dark chocolate instead of thinking about it for two days," she advises.

After all, deprivation only leads to out-of-control cravings, which can result in out-of-control eating. Better to indulge healthfully with one of Chef Devin's S'mores Protein Pudding "Pie" (page 208) than to suddenly stare into an empty pie tin that, just a few minutes earlier, contained a full-size chocolate cream pie.

As for taste? We'll let you be the judge. But after you try the Chocolate Banana "Ice Cream" (page 207) or Punched-Up Piña Colada (page 213), we doubt you'll have any reservations about that.

MAKE A DIFFERENCE IN 20 MINUTES
Check, Please!

On date night with your spouse, what's more romantic than splitting a to-die-for dessert at the end of dinner? How about getting cozy with your honey—just 20 minutes of canoodling with your better half can burn about 30 calories. Make that a double and burn 60 . . . and so on. We'll leave the rest to you.

BAKED CHERRIES A LA MO-GURT

It's surprising how yummy and satisfying the simple combination of tart cherries and sweet vanilla yogurt can be. This warm dessert is extra satisfying on a cold winter's night. It's slightly reminiscent of cherry pie a la mode, yet saves you hours on the treadmill—always a plus!

Canola oil spray (propellant free)

1 can (14.5 ounces) red tart cherries in water, drained*

2 tablespoons whole grain oat flour

1½ tablespoons light agave nectar

2 tablespoons fat-free, preferably fruit juice–sweetened vanilla yogurt

Preheat the oven to 400°F. Lightly mist two 3½"-diameter (½-cup capacity) ramekins with the canola oil spray.

In a small mixing bowl, gently stir the cherries, flour, and agave until well combined, being careful not to crush the cherries (this would add excess liquid to the mixture). Divide the mixture evenly among the ramekins.

Bake for 17 to 19 minutes, or until the cherries resemble pie filling. Cool for 2 minutes, then top each with 1 tablespoon of the yogurt. Serve immediately.

Makes 2 servings

Per serving: 147 calories, 3 g protein, 34 g carbohydrates (25 g sugar), < 1 g fat, trace saturated fat, 0 mg cholesterol, 3 g fiber, 11 mg sodium

*Be sure to check the label. Avoid cherries that contain added sweeteners.

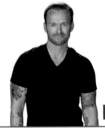

Biggest Loser Trainer Tip: Bob Harper

It's okay to indulge as long as you do it intelligently. Many items such as sorbet come in individual portions. So don't be tempted to buy the entire pint, when a couple of bites is all you need. And remember to always write those calories down in your food journal and work them off when you go to the gym.

CHOCOLATE RASPBERRY DREAMERS

I'll admit that I had no idea what to call this dessert. The chocolate is lighter than a pudding but not as fluffy as a mousse and certainly didn't resemble anything fudgy. But it is delicious and satisfying, especially given how few calories it has (not to mention the 10 grams of fiber). On those nights (and afternoons) when you dream about having a sweet, chocolatey snack, this one fits the bill!

---

1 cup all-natural fat-free cottage cheese

3 tablespoons 100% fruit raspberry spread

2 tablespoons cocoa powder

4 cups fresh raspberries

2 tablespoons natural 70% cocoa mini dark chocolate chunks

To the jar of a blender, add the cottage cheese, fruit spread, and cocoa powder. Blend on high until smooth, turning off the blender intermittently to scrape down the sides. Transfer the mixture to a resealable plastic container and refrigerate for 1 hour, or until chilled.

Divide the raspberries evenly among 4 martini glasses or to-go cups with lids. Spoon one-quarter of the chocolate mixture (about ¼ cup) over each and top with ½ tablespoon of chocolate chunks.

Makes 4 servings

Per serving: **179 calories, 9 g protein, 31 g carbohydrates (17 g sugar), 3 g fat, 2 g saturated fat, 3 mg cholesterol, 10 g fiber, 216 mg sodium**

> ### ⟩⟩⟩ TAKE IT TO GO! ⟩⟩⟩
>
> This is a simple dessert for when you're on the go. To keep the raspberries fresh, pack them separately in a resealable plastic bag and spoon the chocolate mixture into a resealable container. Of course, you'll want to keep it all on ice or refrigerated until you're ready to enjoy.

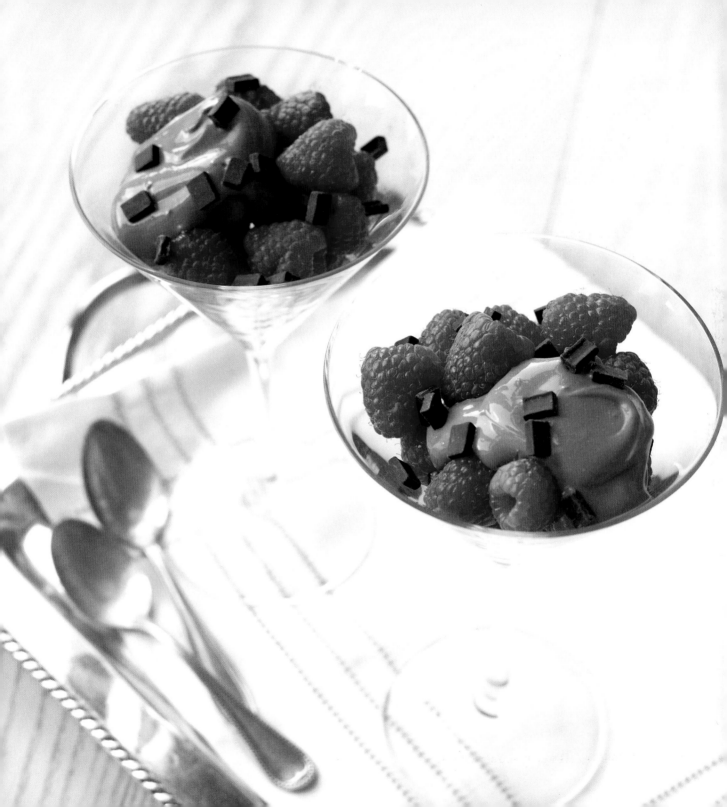

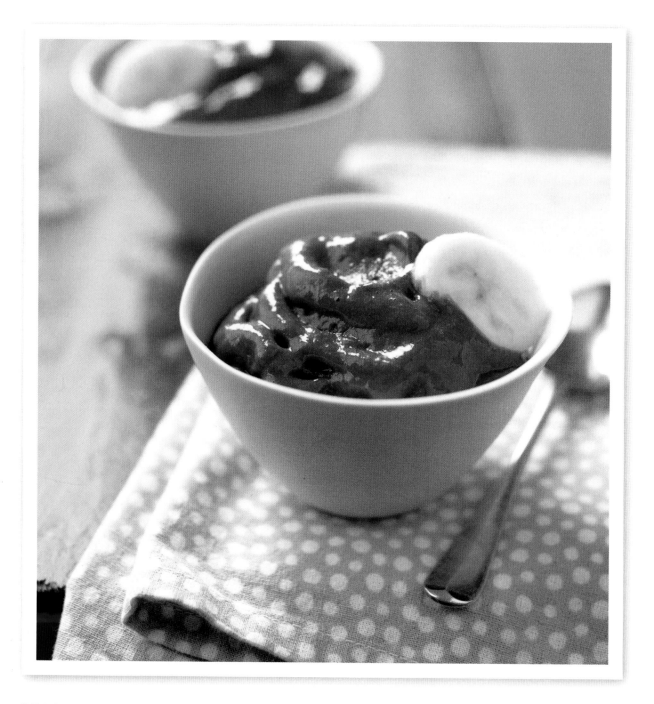

CHOCOLATE BANANA "ICE CREAM"

Be sure not to use overly ripe bananas when you make this dessert. While those are great for baked goods like banana breads and muffins, it's better to use slightly firm bananas for this recipe (and for smoothies). Also, note that the serving size may vary slightly depending on the size of the bananas you use. If you don't have frozen bananas on hand, cut fresh ripe bananas into 1" pieces, place them in an airtight container, and freeze for at least 1 to 2 hours.

2 medium frozen bananas

1 scoop (17 grams) Biggest Loser All Natural Chocolate Deluxe Protein Supplement, or 50 calories' worth of another chocolate protein powder

1 tablespoon all-natural cocoa powder

Remove the bananas from the freezer and cut into 1" pieces. Add the bananas, protein powder, and cocoa powder to the bowl of a food processor fitted with a chopping blade. Process until completely smooth, pausing if necessary to scrape down the sides of the bowl. Continue processing for 1 minute longer, or until it is aerated and fluffy (be careful not to overprocess, or it will begin to liquefy). Divide the ice cream evenly among 2 small dessert bowls. Serve immediately.

Makes 2 (heaping ½-cup) servings

Per serving: 145 calories, 5 g protein, 35 g carbohydrates (22 g sugar), <1 g fat, trace saturated fat, 10 mg cholesterol, 8 g fiber, 28 mg sodium

Joe Mitchell SEASON 12

To satisfy my sweet tooth, I love combining Greek yogurt with Truvía and strawberries. Just throw it all in a bowl and mix it up. It curbs my desire for ice cream!

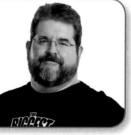

S'MORES PROTEIN PUDDING "PIE"

My friend Allison, who is a health coach, mentioned one day that she spikes pudding with protein powder to make pudding pies. It was seconds before I asked her if I could "borrow" her idea!

If you're not familiar with ricemellow crème, it's very similar to marshmallow crème but a bit less dense, and it's sweetened with natural brown rice syrup instead of corn syrup. Look for it in natural food stores.

---

2 tablespoons whole grain, crunchy, high-fiber, low-sugar cereal (I used Kashi 7 Whole Grain Nuggets)

2 (4-ounce) cups all-natural, chocolate pudding, preferably agave-sweetened (I used Potter Family Organics Chocolate Pudding)

1 scoop (17 grams) Biggest Loser All Natural Chocolate Deluxe Protein Supplement (or 50 calories' worth of other chocolate protein powder)*

4 tablespoons all-natural marshmallow crème (I used Suzanne's Ricemellow Creme)

Divide the cereal between two 3½"-diameter (½-cup capacity) ramekins.

In a small bowl, stir together the pudding and protein powder until well combined. Spoon half over the cereal in each ramekin.

Dollop the top of each with 2 tablespoons of the marshmallow crème. Serve immediately.

Makes 2 servings

Per serving: 158 calories, 9 g protein, 30 g carbohydrates (14 g sugar), 1 g fat, trace saturated fat, 10 mg cholesterol, 6 g fiber, 146 mg sodium

If you don't have protein powder, this recipe is just as delicious without it. If you skip it, it just won't have as much fiber or protein.

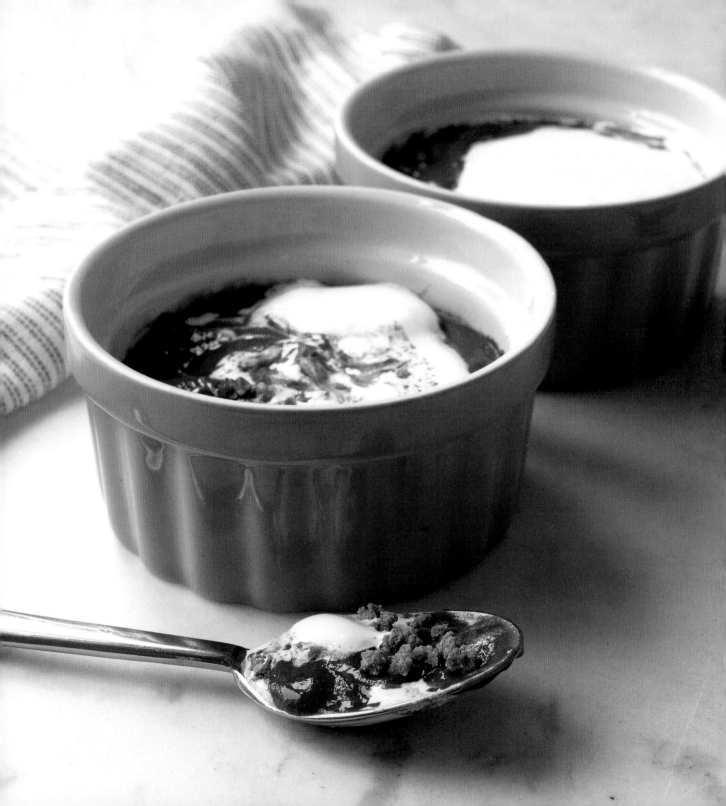

MMMM . . . MONKEY TRAIL MIX

Like granola, trail mix is one of those tricky "healthy" foods. Yes, there can be a lot of health benefits in the nuts (if they're dry-roasted) and in unsweetened dried fruit. But granola and trail mix also tend to be very calorie-dense, so portion control is key. Here, I've created an alternative to traditional trail mixes that your kids—and the kid inside of you—are likely to love.

---

1 cup all-natural crunchy corn peanut butter cereal (I used Mother's Peanut Butter Bumpers)

1 cup all-natural chocolate and peanut butter puffs cereal (I used Barbara's Peanut Butter and Chocolate Puffins)

⅓ cup (½ ounce) freeze-dried unsweetened bananas

2 tablespoons natural 70% cocoa mini dark chocolate chunks

2 tablespoons dry-roasted, lightly salted almonds

In a medium bowl, mix the cereals, bananas, chocolate chunks, and almonds until well combined. Divide the trail mix evenly among 4 snack-size resealable plastic bags. Serve immediately or store the bags in a medium resealable plastic container.*

Makes 4 (heaping ½-cup) servings

Per serving: **139** calories, **3 g** protein, **22 g** carbohydrates (9 g sugar), **6 g** fat, **2 g** saturated fat, **0 mg** cholesterol, **3 g** fiber, **108 mg** sodium

Be sure to store the snack-size bags in a resealable plastic container, as most resealable plastic bags will not keep the mix from going stale.

>>> TAKE IT TO GO! >>>

This is the perfect to-go snack. Just measure out individual servings and place them in resealable baggies. Tuck them into lunch boxes, backpacks, purses, or desk drawers for healthy snacking on the go.

WATERMELON COCKTAIL

This simple dessert is all about the presentation. After measuring the balsamic glaze, it's best to transfer it from a measuring teaspoon to a serving teaspoon to do the drizzling. It's much easier to create a pretty drizzle pattern that way. Another option is to transfer the glaze to a small squirt bottle, to ensure you create even lines.

1 cup seedless ½" watermelon cubes (5¾ ounces)

1 teaspoon natural balsamic glaze (get one with no added sugar)

Fresh mint leaf, for garnish (optional)

Place the watermelon cubes in a chilled martini glass. Drizzle the glaze over the top of the watermelon. Garnish with mint, if desired. Serve immediately.

Makes 1 serving

Per serving: 57 calories, <1 g protein, 14 g carbohydrates (12 g sugar), trace fat, trace saturated fat, 0 mg cholesterol, <1 g fiber, 3 mg sodium

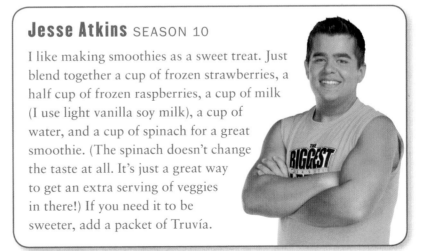

Jesse Atkins SEASON 10

I like making smoothies as a sweet treat. Just blend together a cup of frozen strawberries, a half cup of frozen raspberries, a cup of milk (I use light vanilla soy milk), a cup of water, and a cup of spinach for a great smoothie. (The spinach doesn't change the taste at all. It's just a great way to get an extra serving of veggies in there!) If you need it to be sweeter, add a packet of Truvía.

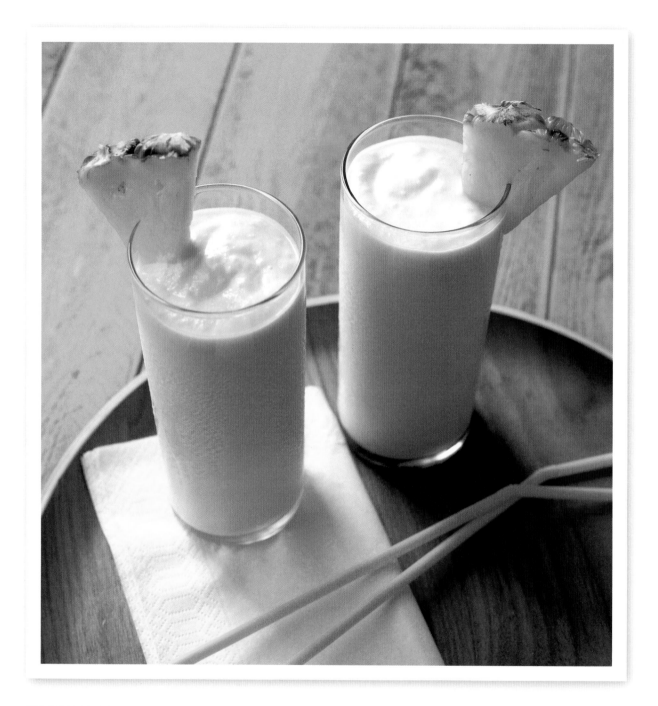

PUNCHED-UP PIÑA COLADA

Most cocktails contain a lot of calories and empty carbohydrates. Here I've replaced calorie-dense coconut crème with light coconut milk, and used frozen pineapple chunks and dried egg whites to thicken the drink. The frozen pineapple retains more nutrients than the sugar-sweetened pineapple juice typically used in a piña colada, and the egg whites add about 5 grams of protein. In the end, you save a whopping 307 calories, 13 grams of fat, and 12 grams of saturated fat over a typical same-size piña colada!

½ cup light coconut milk

8 ice cubes

3 cups frozen pineapple chunks

2 tablespoons 100% dried egg whites (I used Deb-El Just Whites), optional

3 tablespoons light rum

2 pineapple wedges for garnish (optional)

To the jar of a blender with an ice crush setting, add the coconut milk, ice cubes, pineapple chunks, egg whites (if desired), and rum. Blend on high just until the mixture is smooth. Divide it between 2 chilled Collins glasses or other tall, thin glasses. Garnish with the pineapple wedges, if desired, and serve immediately with straws and/or drink umbrellas.

Makes 2 servings

Per serving (with egg whites): **219 calories, 6 g protein, 33 g carbohydrates (23 g sugar), 4 g fat, 3 g saturated fat, 0 mg cholesterol, 3 g fiber, 83 mg sodium**

Per serving (without egg whites): **204 calories, 1 g protein, 33 g carbohydrates (23 g sugar), 4 g fat, 3 g saturated fat, 0 mg cholesterol, 3 g fiber, 8 mg sodium**

Brendon Donovan SEASON 10

My favorite sweet treat on the Ranch was crushed strawberries, blueberries, and peaches with a sprinkling of Truvía, stevia, or agave nectar.

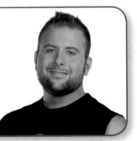

Acknowledgments

Devin Alexander

I think I may be the luckiest girl in the world to get to continually be a part of the *Biggest Loser* family. With five cookbooks in partnership, I not only get to hear from and interface with amazing fans of the show who have been inspired and inspire, I also have the honor of working with some of the most amazing professionals in the business.

The whole team at Rodale rocks, particularly: Julie Will, who happens to be a brilliant editor *and* who I'm going to miss like crazy if our "three seconds later" partnership ever ends; Pam Krauss, who came in and made phase two of this book a snap; Production Editor Nancy Bailey, who makes sure the trains run on time; Designer Christina Gaugler, who made the pages look so enticing with the help of Killer Photographer Mitch Mandell; Publisher Extraordinaire Karen Rinaldi; and Publicity Goddesses Emily Weber and Yelena Nesbit.

To the super-cool Dr. Michael Dansinger, who totally "gets it." He's extremely professional and knowledgeable, yet allows me to be the voice of healthy decadence as needed.

To the ultimate coordinator Edwin Karapetian. To Reveille's Vice President of Brand Development and Production Chad Bennett, who's worked with me on every book and whom I absolutely adore beyond words. And to uber-cool Executive Producer Todd Lubin—you're my new hero!

To the producers and executives of *The Biggest Loser*, particularly Howard Owens of Reveille, who made me the happiest girl ever when they first invited me into the *Biggest Loser* family. To Kim Niemi, Neysa Siefert, and Joni Camacho from NBCUniversal, and to Dave Broome and Yong Yam from 25/7 Productions, who are simply the best!

To Bob Harper and Jillian Michaels for embracing me and my work over the years, and to new "recruits" Anna Kournikova and Dolvett Quince. To every *Biggest Loser* contestant who spent time in my kitchen and let me visit theirs, inspiring so many of my creations.

To Sara Wing and the team at Cabot's, who provided plenty of their insanely great 75 percent reduced-fat Cheddar cheese. And to Rachel Litner and Mary Rodgers of Cuisinart for sending me the coolest blender/food processor combo and kitchen scales when mine freaked out right before deadline.

To my WME agents Suzanne Lyons and Ivo Fischer, for their support and determination on my behalf—woo hoo! To Becca Oliver, for making a difference "with one phone call." To Lauren Zander and Rebecca Bent of the Handel Group, who've helped turn my most recent dreams into realities. And to my sister, Leslie Simone, also of the Handel Group, for constantly growing with me and for just being you!

And a very special thanks to the incredible team in my kitchen as well as my recipe testers—Stephanie Farrell, Alexandra Gudmundsson, Jordan Rebecca Harris, Miriam Heath, and Allison Samon. You save my life daily, and I couldn't have done it without you!

Julie Will

Big, heartfelt thanks to the multitalented Chad Bennett and the rest of *The Biggest Loser* and Reveille family: It's such a pleasure to work with you guys. To all of my friends and colleagues at Rodale, especially Karen Rinaldi, Pam Krauss, Nancy Bailey, Chris Gaugler, Melissa Roberson, Yelena Nesbit, and the amazing Marie Crousillat: Thank you for your shrewd intellect and limitless patience. And to Devin Alexander: You are the hardest working, most diligent author I know—thanks for your great, creative content—and for letting me sample your recipes.

And lastly, to my family and friends: I don't know why you put up with me, but I am so lucky, and grateful, that you do. Thank you.

Index

Underscored page references indicate sidebars and tables. **Boldface** references indicate photographs.

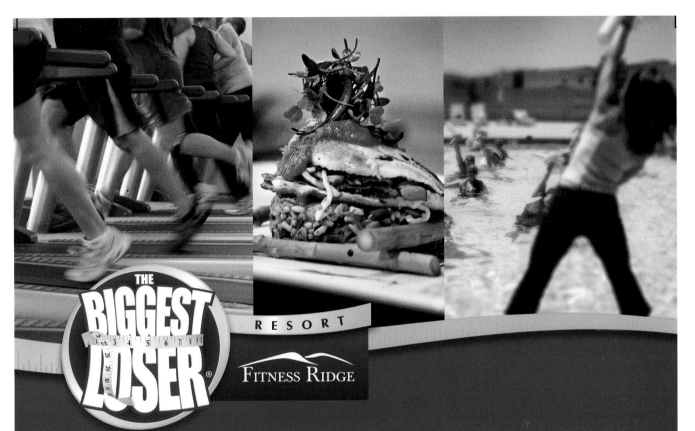

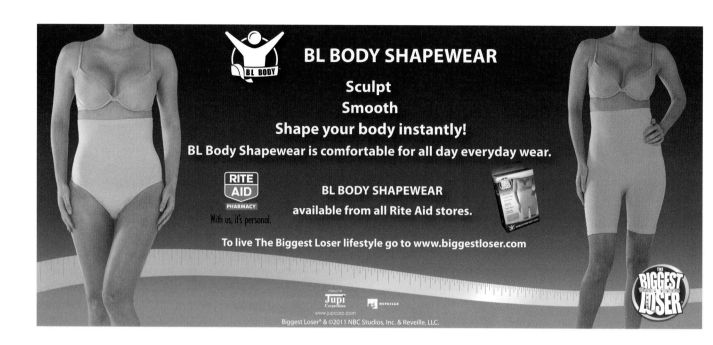

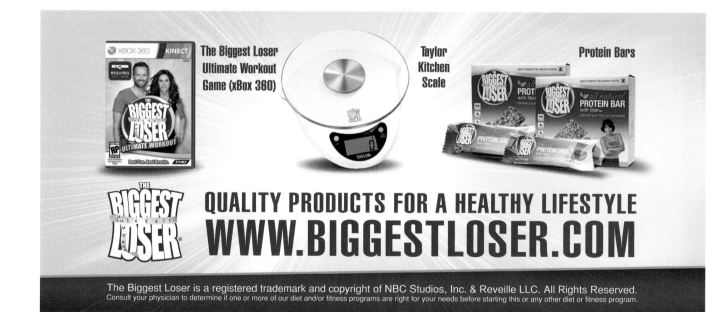

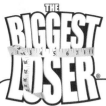
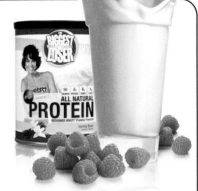
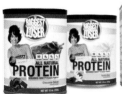 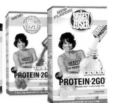
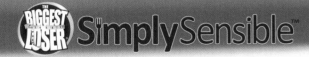

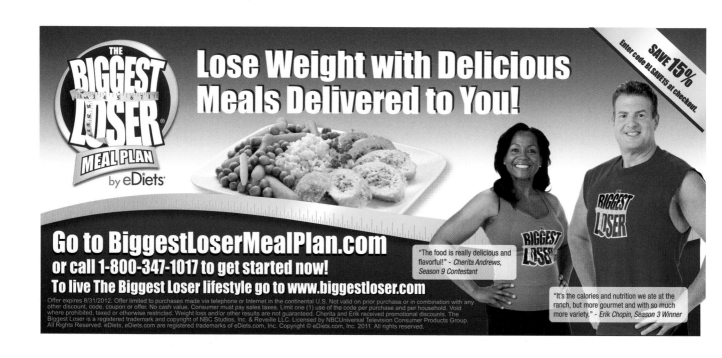
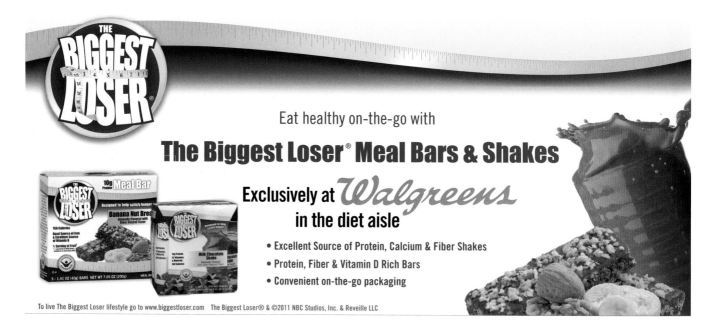

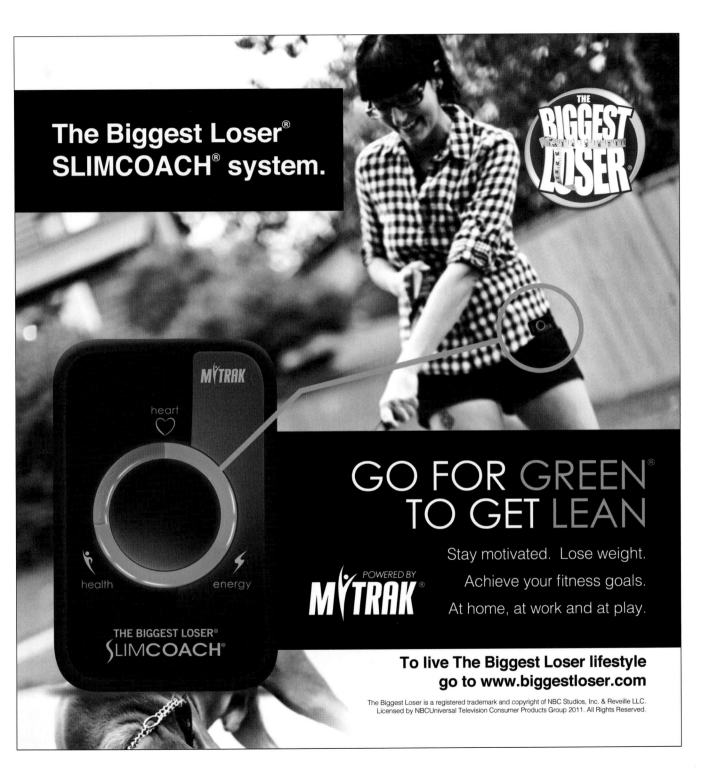

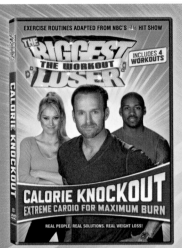
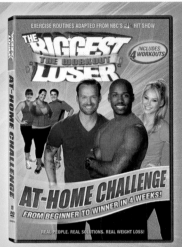
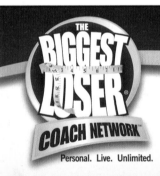
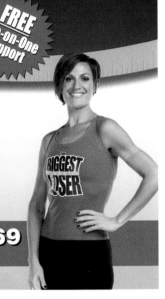

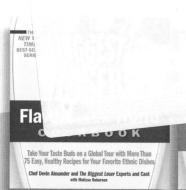
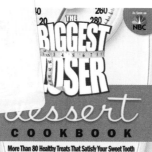
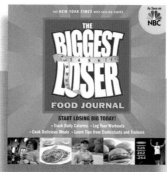
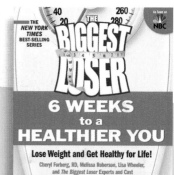
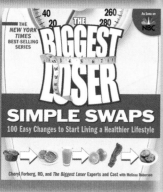
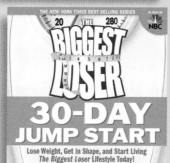
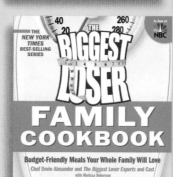
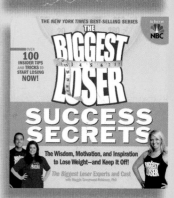
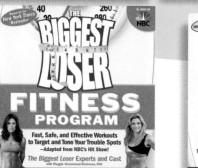
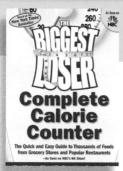
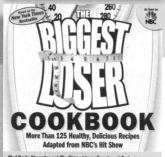
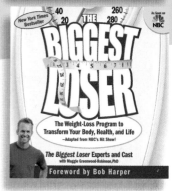
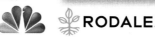

SERIOUS ABOUT LOSING WEIGHT?
JOIN THE CLUB!

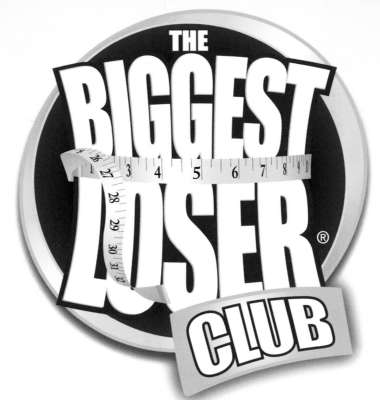

You're just a click away from a slimmer, healthier new you!

Why take your weight loss and healthy living goals online with The Biggest Loser Club? For starters, you'll find: Hundreds of additional recipes ■ Tips and feedback from the trainers and show contestants ■ Support from our team of experts and other members ■ Customized meal plans, suited to your tastes ■ Tools to keep you on track toward your calorie targets ■ Automatic shopping lists ■ Individualized exercise plans based on your fitness level and goals ■ Convenient 24/7 access

Go online TODAY for your FREE diet profile!
Visit www.biggestloserclub.com/cookbook